# Hypertension

**Michael Schachter** BSc (Hons), MBBS, FRCP
Senior Lecturer in Clinical Pharmacology and Therapeutics
Faculty of Medicine, Imperial College, London

Honorary Consultant Physician
St Mary's Hospital NHS Trust, London

**David Monkman** MBBS, MRCP, DRCOG, FPCert
General Practitioner
East Barnet Health Centre, Barnet, Hertfordshire, UK

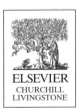

ELSEVIER
CHURCHILL
LIVINGSTONE

EDINBURGH   LONDON   NEW YORK   OXFORD   PHILADELPHIA   ST LOUIS   SYDNEY   TORONTO   2004

# ELSEVIER
## CHURCHILL
## LIVINGSTONE

The right of Michael Schachter and David Monkman to be identified as authors of this work has been asserted by them in accordance with the Copyright, Designs and Patents Act 1988

First published 2004

ISBN 0443 074704

British Library Cataloguing in Publication Data
A catalogue record for this book is available from the British Library

Library of Congress Cataloging in Publication Data
A catalog record for this book is available from the Library of Congress

Notice
Medical knowledge is constantly changing. Standard safety precautions must be followed, but as new reasearch and clinical experience broaden our knowledge, changes in treatment and drug therapy may become necessary or appropriate. Readers are advised to check the most current product information provided by the manufacturer of each drug to be administered to verify the recommended dose, the method and duration of administration, and contraindications. It is the responsibility of the practitioner, relying on experience and knowledge of the patient, to determine dosages and the best treatment for each individual patient. Neither the Publisher nor the authors assumes any liability for any injury and/or damage to persons or property arising from this publication.

*The Publisher*

Front cover image of hypertensive retinopathy reproduced with kind permission of Gregory YH Lip, from Lip et al. Fundal changes in malignant hypertension. J Hum Hypertens 1997;11:395–6. © 1997 Stockton Press.

Front cover image of aortogram showing renal artery lesions reproduced with permission from Hallett et al. Comprehensive Vascular and Endovascular Surgery. Mosby, 2004.

Printed in China

The
Publisher's
policy is to use
**paper manufactured
from sustainable forests**

# Contents

# Preface

Anyone involved in primary care is going to spend a large percentage of their professional time managing hypertension. This problem is growing and will continue to do so, at least in part, because of the moving goalposts. Soon we will all be hypertensives or latent hypertensives: a slight exaggeration but one that reflects increasing stringency in defining "normal" blood pressure.

This short book is intended to help deal with this effectively. As much as anything it becomes a challenge in communicating with our patients in a situation where we may want to persuade them to commit to a lifetime of medication, perhaps 30 years or more, after we have made the diagnosis. We need to persuade them, and indeed ourselves, that this is worth doing. If the health professionals are not convinced, the patients surely will not be. The fact is that it is worthwhile, but we must also make it as tolerable as we can by using the most suitable medication at the lowest possible doses.

Hypertension is unusual in many ways, not least because we have so many treatments for the condition without really understanding its underlying cause. But, at least, we are much luckier than our predecessors in having a menu to choose from. A large part of this short book deals with how best to choose from that menu. It also tries to provide a framework for understanding current ideas about this condition and for assessing our patients. Perhaps one of the key messages can be summarized simply: do not over investigate. It wastes time for the patient and for us, and of course wastes money.

What this book does *not* do is substitute for the extensive and detailed guidelines prepared and published by experts in the UK, Europe and the USA. They are referred to throughout the book and are readily accessible online. Still less is it an encyclopaedia of hypertension, several of which are in preparation (by others). However, we do hope that it will be a useful concise guide to most of the hypertension-related problems that are likely to occur in non-specialist practice. Although we have tried to present consensus views wherever possible it is likely that the authors' views and prejudices do surface in places. We hope they are clearly sign-posted and not too obtrusive!

**Michael Schachter**
Senior Lecturer in Clinical Pharmacology and Therapeutics
Faculty of Medicine, Imperial College, London, and
Honorary Consultant Physician
St Mary's Hospital NHS Trust, London

**David Monkman**
General Practitioner
East Barnet Health Centre, Barnet, Hertfordshire, UK

# Biographies

**Michael Schachter BSc (Hons), MBBS, FRCP** trained at University College and University College Hospital in London. His main general medical training was at King's College Hospital, obtaining his MRCP, and he subsequently joined the University Department of Neurology as a research registrar. His research was mainly focused on the treatment of Parkinson's disease and narcolepsy, and the clinical pharmacology of the drugs used in these disorders. He then moved to the MRC Unit and University Department of Clinical Pharmacology in Oxford, working on platelet pharmacology and the mechanisms of receptor adaptation during long-term drug therapies. He moved to the then St Mary's Hospital Medical School in 1984 and obtained a British Heart Foundation Senior Research Fellowship working on the role of vascular structural change in hypertension and the underlying biochemical mechanisms. His research interests remain primarily concerned with hypertension and its treatment, as well as the clinical pharmacology of lipid-lowering drugs. He is also interested in problems of errors in drug prescribing and administration and their clinical implications. He participates in a large hypertension/cardiovascular risk clinic and currently has a major involvement in the organization of all aspects of undergraduate education in his medical school.

Mike Schachter has over 200 publications in the areas mentioned and has also written, edited and contributed to books on hypertension, lipids and the side effects of drugs, as well as being a member of the editorial board of several journals.

**David Monkman MBBS, MRCP, DRCOG, FPCert** qualified at the Royal Free Hospital in 1981. After completing general medical training and paediatrics, he took his MRCP in 1985. He then spent two and a half years in training as a haematologist before deciding to go into general practice. He has been a GP in North London for over 15 years, and during his time in general practice has developed a keen interest in the management and prevention of cardiovascular disease. He is a Deanery tutor and is a PEC member of his local PCT. He has been a GP representative of guideline groups both at a local and national level.

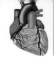
## Introduction

Sir George Pickering, one of the founders of British hypertension research, commented that the problem with clinicians is they can only count to two. Of course many of us can do better than that, what he meant was that doctors are used to binary situations: does the patient have a particular disease or not. Some of his critics proposed that hypertension too could be considered in this way: however, his view and one that is now generally accepted, is that it cannot.

*" The risk associated with blood pressure is linear over a wide range of values "*

There is a distribution of blood pressure among all populations and hypertension describes a proportion of that population. The risk associated with blood pressure is linear over a wide range of values either for systolic or diastolic measurements, so that the concept of normal blood pressure has become more elusive (Figures 1 and 2).[1,2]

**Fig. 1 Prevalence of hypertension by different cut-off points.** Based on data in the UK.

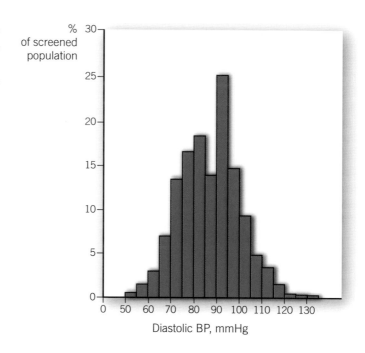

As we shall see, the proportion of people considered to be hypertensive has been increasing in the last 30 years largely because our definitions of hypertension have become increasingly rigorous with progressively lower thresholds. Ultimately we are always left with a question of judgement, whether we use blood pressure as a stand-alone criterion for deciding whether or not to intervene, or whether it is incorporated into a global risk assessment. These issues are further complicated by

*" The concept of normal blood pressure has become more elusive "*

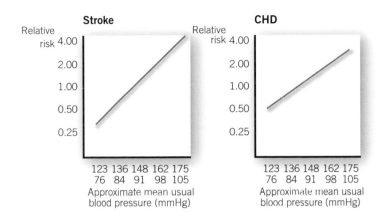

**Fig. 2 Blood pressure and relative risk of stroke and CHD.**

Reproduced from Collins R, MacMahon S. Blood pressure, antihypertensive drug treatment and risk of stroke and coronary heart disease. *Br Med Bull* 1994;50:272–98, by permission of Oxford University Press.

differences of emphasis on systolic and diastolic blood pressures, though these are closer to resolution. Once we have decided that a patient needs some sort of therapeutic intervention, with drugs or otherwise, we have also been confronted with increasingly stringent targets for blood pressure control, while being told that we have been ineffective in achieving the previous targets! Yet it now seems probable that even the well-treated hypertensive patient, with pressure very close to current targets, is still at a disadvantage in terms of survival and cardiovascular events when followed over a period of over 20 years.[3] Even so, progress in detecting and treating hypertension, as well as in promoting public awareness that it is a problem, has certainly been taking place and is continuing.

Hypertension then is more difficult than it looks from every angle, even without considering (as by and large we will not) the contentious issues concerning the cause of so-called essential hypertension, which constitutes 90–95% of the cases seen in most clinical populations. We hope that this book will be helpful for doctors and nurses in primary care who look after the great majority of patients with raised blood pressure. Although the body of knowledge about this condition is now dauntingly large there are, as the readers will note, many times when we simply do not know how best to manage a clinical problem. This is not *always* due to the author's ignorance! Please note that we have not referenced every single statement. This would produce something much more extensive and elaborate than is intended here and we believe would not be especially welcome to most of our readers.

*We have been confronted with increasingly stringent targets for blood pressure control*

*Essential hypertension constitutes 90–95% of the cases seen in most clinical populations*

## Hypertension and ageing populations

It is a cliché that Western populations are ageing, and it also happens to be true. This is the inevitable consequence of low birth rates and greater longevity. It means that in most such societies about 20% of the population will be older than 65 years well before the middle of the 21st century. This will mean a steadily growing number of hypertensive patients who will need to be at least assessed and probably treated. As a result hypertension is among the most important public health issues in Western societies and in fact in the world as a whole.[4] Conversely, societies in the former Soviet bloc appear to have experienced significant declines in life expectancy, especially among men, but these too are largely linked to coronary artery disease with hypertension being one of the identifiable risk factors.

> *Hypertension is among the most important public health issues in Western societies*

## Relationship to other cardiovascular risk factors

It has become a truism that we can only account for about half the cases of coronary heart disease on the basis of currently recognized risk factors. A truism perhaps but not actually true. More careful analysis of the data suggests that we can at least partly predict most cases of cardiovascular disease on the basis of established factors, including hypertension. But it is clear that there are significant variations in the pattern of the risk factors and their relative importance both in individuals and in specific ethnic groups. For instance, a well-recognized health problem in the UK is the high incidence of premature disease in individuals, especially men, of South Asian origin. Here it is evident that dyslipidaemia, especially low HDL cholesterol, is of particular importance and this often forms part of the so-called metabolic syndrome including dyslipidaemia, insulin resistance or overt diabetes, and hypertension. In all circumstances we can see that risk factors interact strongly, often in synergistic or multiplicative ways. Global risk assessment, incorporating at least:

> *We can at least partly predict most cases of cardiovascular disease on the basis of established factors, including hypertension*

- age
- gender
- blood pressure, systolic or diastolic
- diabetes, absent or present rather than severity
- lipid profile ideally both LDL and HDL, possibly also triglycerides
- family history, in some models,

can provide a useful guide to risk based on the Framingham, Munster and other studies (see Ref. 5 for example of risk charts) (for fuller list see Figure 3). But it has to be recognized that the calculations may not be appropriate for all populations. It has also to be acknowledged, however, that blood pressure is still very often seen as a stand-alone problem and clinical practice as well as official guidelines are based on the assumption that some levels of blood pressure always require treatment regardless of the presence of other risk factors or of existing target organ damage.

> *Blood pressure is still very often seen as a stand-alone problem*

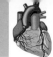

| Risk factors for cardiovascular disease |
| --- |
| **Modifiable risk factors** |
| • Smoking |
| • Dyslipidaemia |
|    – raised LDL-cholesterol |
|    – low HDL-cholesterol |
|    – raised triglycerides |
| • Raised blood pressure |
| • Diabetes mellitus/metabolic syndrome |
| • Obesity (BMI > 30) |
| • Dietary factors |
| • Thrombogenic factors |
| • Lack of exercise |
| • Excess alcohol consumption |
| • Increased homocysteine levels? |
| • Raised c-reactive protein |
| **Non-modifiable risk factors** |
| • Personal history of CHD |
| • Family history of CHD |
| • Age |
| • Gender |

Fig. 3 Risk factors for cardiovascular disease.

# Definition and epidemiology
## Changing criteria for defining hypertension

From today's clinical perspective the inclusion criteria for the early hypertension trials seem quite horrific: not many people would now exclude individuals with diastolic blood pressure over 120mmHg from treatment! In the 1960s some trials did exactly that, for several reasons. First, the range of drugs then available was very limited and generally not well tolerated. Second, risk factors like blood pressure and cholesterol (and perhaps now homocysteine) follow a recognizable "lifecycle" (Figure 4).

There are usually no easy answers to the last point of the "lifecycle", as we know. Nonetheless, the pattern is recognizable to everyone involved in managing cardiovascular disease and more especially in trying to prevent it. One implication of this process is that the efficacy and acceptability of available treatments will have a major impact on the definitions of hypertension. One is always reluctant to aim at unattainable clinical targets. The most recent of the widely accepted definitions of hypertension originates from the United States

*"The efficacy and acceptability of available treatments will have a major impact on the definitions of hypertension"*

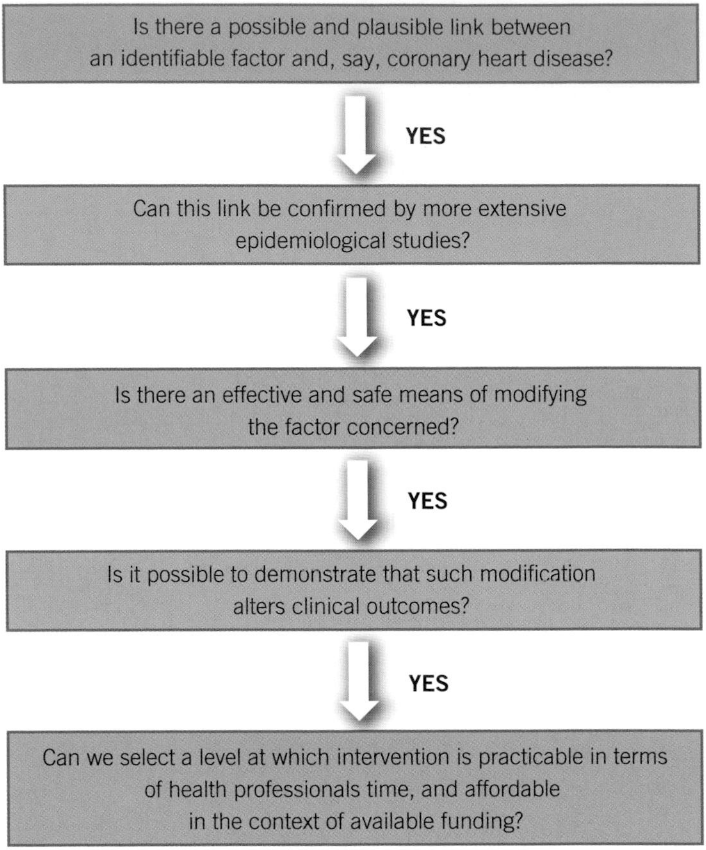

**Fig. 4 The "lifecycle" of risk factors.**

Is there a possible and plausible link between an identifiable factor and, say, coronary heart disease?

**YES**

Can this link be confirmed by more extensive epidemiological studies?

**YES**

Is there an effective and safe means of modifying the factor concerned?

**YES**

Is it possible to demonstrate that such modification alters clinical outcomes?

**YES**

Can we select a level at which intervention is practicable in terms of health professionals time, and affordable in the context of available funding?

> **❝ Optimal blood pressure appears to be at systolic pressure of 115–120mmHg ❞**

Joint National Committee of Prevention and Treatment of High Blood Pressure (JNC7)[6] and from the Joint European Society of Cardiology/European Society of Hypertension guidelines,[5] published almost simultaneously. As Figure 5 shows, this approach incorporates the idea of high normal blood pressure: in fact the JNC7 reports regard systolic blood pressures above 120mmHg as "pre-hypertensive". Of course, optimal blood pressure appears to be at systolic pressure of 115–120mmHg, hardly a realistic target for large populations using current therapeutics, or anything that is likely to be available in the near future. It has been said, perhaps cynically, that the main purpose of guidelines in hypertension is to focus attention on the previous set of guidelines and this may be near the truth, as we will see when considering what is actually achieved in clinical practice.

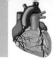

| Category | Systolic (mmHg) | Diastolic (mmHg) |
|---|---|---|
| Optimal | <120 | <80 |
| Normal | 120 – 129 | 80 –84 |
| High normal | 130 – 139 | 85 – 89 |
| Grade 1 hypertension (mild) | 140 – 159 | 90 – 99 |
| Grade 2 hypertension (moderate) | 160 – 179 | 100 – 109 |
| Grade 3 hypertension (severe) | ≥ 180 | ≥ 110 |
| Isolated systolic hypertension | ≥ 140 | < 80 |

Fig. 5 Classification of blood pressure based on current European guidelines.

## Systolic and diastolic blood pressure: which matters more?

Until recently it almost went without saying, both among health professionals and the public, that diastolic blood pressure is more important than systolic. Most of the pioneering blood pressure trials used diastolic pressure as their main parameter. More recently, emphasis has shifted towards systolic pressure or to pulse pressure as the best indicator of prognosis. This has been based partly on epidemiological data and partly on the results of clinical trials. Some researchers have focused on the importance of central (aortic) blood pressure rather than that measured at the brachial artery. There are non-invasive methods of estimating this but the methodology is controversial and certainly is not available for routine clinical use.

*"Most of the pioneering blood pressure trials used diastolic pressure as their main parameter"*

The current consensus on this difficult issue can be summarized as follows:[5,6]

- diastolic blood pressure may be the best indicator of overall risk in individuals below the age of 50, especially women
- from the age of 50 to 60 or 65 there is little difference between systolic, diastolic and pulse pressures as markers of risk; it is possible that a mean of the two may actually be best
- above this age systolic and pulse pressure are clearly superior.
Specific issues concerning ageing and changes in blood pressure will be considered in the next section.

There are also significant practical considerations relating to this question. The diastolic pressure may be more difficult to measure accurately, whether manually with auscultation or with electronic

*«Systolic pressure can almost always be measured accurately by auscultation, palpation or electronically»*

automatic or semi-automatic devices. The total disappearance of the pulse (Korotkoff phase 5, see section on measurement) may not be detectable in some individuals, or may only be detected rather imprecisely, while systolic pressure can almost always be measured accurately by auscultation, palpation or electronically.

### Blood pressure and ageing: isolated systolic hypertension[7]

As has already been noted, in most societies blood pressure, and therefore the incidence of hypertension, rises with age (Figure 6). Most

Fig. 6 Schematic representation of change of blood pressure with age in western populations.

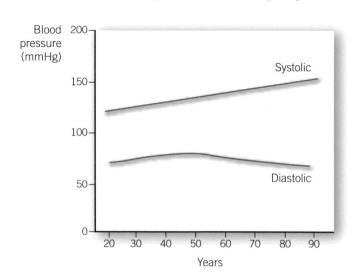

*«Most people will be classified as hypertensive if they live long enough»*

people will be classified as hypertensive if they live long enough: it has recently been estimated that if an individual is normotensive at the age of 55 the likelihood of developing hypertension later in life is approximately 90%, using current definitions. This may appear to be an inevitable part of ageing but this is almost certainly not the case. There are societies, although decreasing in number, where this rise in blood pressure hardly occurs at all or only to a very limited extent. In most places though we can expect *systolic* blood pressure to increase steadily with age. By contrast, *diastolic* blood pressure tends to decline from about the age of 50–60 years. As a consequence, most hypertension in those older than 60 years (as much as 75–80% in this age group) is characterized as *isolated systolic hypertension* (see Figure 5 for classification of hypertension).

In the UK the upper limit for the systolic pressure has been set at 160mmHg,[8] though this is reduced to 140mmHg in patients where other risk factors are present, especially in younger patients. But a systolic pressure of 160mmHg should usually warrant intervention even if no other problem is apparent (see below). Several trials have now demonstrated the benefits of lowering blood pressure in these patients, at least up to the age of about 80 years: a trial (HYVET) is in progress to assess the value of treatment in patients older than this.[9] However, it is interesting to note that in these very elderly individuals blood pressure that would generally be regarded as optimal (<130/80mmHg approximately) is in fact associated with a *poor* prognosis, presumably because these low pressures reflect subnormal left ventricular function or other serious illness, such as malignancy.

*“The factors regulating blood pressure are in principle very straightforward”*

But if, as is usually the case, the systolic pressure (at least) rises with age, what is the underlying cause and mechanism? How much does this differ from the causes and mechanisms relevant to younger individuals?

## Causes of hypertension

As everyone will remember from their physiology lectures, the factors regulating blood pressure are in principle very straightforward: they are cardiac output and peripheral resistance. In most, but as we will see not all, cases of established hypertension there is increased peripheral resistance as the immediate cause of raised blood pressure. The Swedish physiologist Bjorn Folkow and Tony Lever, the former head of the MRC Blood Pressure Unit in Glasgow, evolved the scheme shown in Figure 7 over a period of some 20 years.[10] It does of course

**Fig. 7 The Folkow-Lever hypothesis.** AII = angiotensin II; IGF = insulin-like growth factor; many other candidates may be relevant.

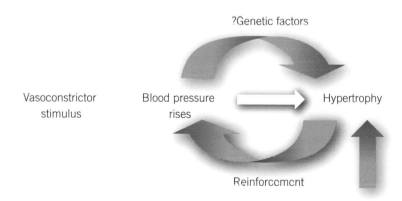

?Genetic factors

Vasoconstrictor stimulus

Blood pressure rises

Hypertrophy

Reinforcement

Growth factors (?AII, IGF etc.)

beg the immediate question: what actually initiates this process, in other words why is there vasoconstriction in the first place? Here we have few certainties, though this scheme suggests a key role for

> **Direct studies have shown that established hypertension is associated with significant changes in small vessel structure**

angiotensin II. But the Folkow-Lever hypothesis does have other implications. It helps to explain why most cases of secondary hypertension are not cured even if the original cause is removed and it also gives a plausible explanation for the increase in blood pressure seen in most treated patients on drug withdrawal. Direct studies have shown that established hypertension is associated with significant changes in small vessel structure and that these are only partially reversed in the majority of patients, even those with excellent blood pressure control over several years.[11]

The exact nature of these changes is highly controversial and the possibilities are summarized in Figure 8. For obvious reasons it is very

**Fig. 8** Schematic view of changes in small artery/arteriole structure, all leading to increased peripheral resistance and therefore raised blood pressure.

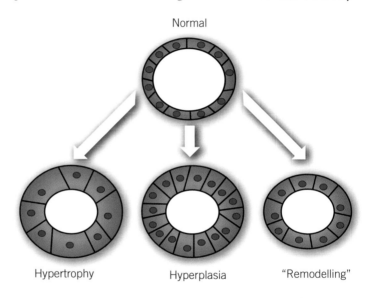

difficult to determine which of these is particularly important in human hypertension, as opposed to animal models. Some researchers have proposed that loss of capillaries (rarefaction) actually makes a larger contribution to the increased peripheral resistance than structural change in small arteries and arterioles.

> **In most people hypertension has a multifactorial basis**

## Essential (primary) hypertension

Over the last few years there has been a marked decline in the enthusiasm for complex and lengthy investigations in most hypertensive patients. This reflects the increasing acceptance of the fact that 90–95% of patients will fall within the rather unsatisfactory heading of essential hypertension. Primary hypertension is a better description. One can regard this as a confession of ignorance, which of

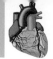

course it is, but also as an acknowledgement that in most people hypertension has a multifactorial basis. While it is not the intention in this book to discuss these issues in any detail, some proposed contributory factors are discussed briefly below.

### Genetics

The genetic basis of hypertension has of course attracted immense interest and indeed funding in the last decade.[12] The likelihood of finding a single gene for essential hypertension is surely negligible but a number of genes have been detected that may have contributory effects on the development of hypertension, albeit each individually to only a modest extent. The genes concerned are involved in the renin-angiotensin system, renal sodium handling and adrenoceptor structure, among others, with the focus moving increasingly towards renal handling of sodium as a, or even the, central problem in essential hypertension. This has long been proposed by investigators such as de Wardener.[13] There has been some progress in linking this classical physiological approach with genetics in the investigation of salt responsiveness. It is possible to divide hypertensives and indeed non-hypertensives into two categories:

- those who are *salt-sensitive* and show a significant rise in blood pressure when salt-loaded, and
- individuals who are *salt-insensitive* and lack this response.

There have been some advances in elucidating the molecular and genetic correlates of this difference. It is of particular interest that black hypertensive populations in the UK and USA are generally salt-sensitive.

A more modest ambition, that of genotyping to help predict responses to specific antihypertensive medication, may be more attainable but is still far from practical in clinical practice and may not be worth pursuing for now.[14] Even so, although genomic approaches have been somewhat disappointing so far, especially in relation to the effort expended, it seems highly likely from analysis of familial genetics that a genetic component forms part of a complex picture of interacting defects. Overall, however, we should continue to think of this condition as a complex polygenic one, with a very large environmental component.

### Prenatal factors and socioeconomic status

The work of Barker and his group, among others, has drawn attention to the possible importance of prenatal environmental factors in the aetiology of essential hypertension.[15] They have proposed that babies of low birth weight, presumably subject to intrauterine malnutrition,

*"The likelihood of finding a single gene for essential hypertension is surely negligible"*

*"It is of particular interest that black hypertensive populations in the UK and USA are generally salt-sensitive"*

*"Babies of low birth weight are more likely to develop hypertension in adult life"*

**15**

are more likely to develop hypertension in adult life. This may also apply to diabetes and other chronic illnesses. The potential mechanisms are beyond the scope of this discussion but the epidemiology so far has provided strong, though not unequivocal, support for the hypothesis. These observations may also in part explain why lower socioeconomic class is strongly linked to higher blood pressures and in fact to almost all forms of chronic cardiovascular and other disease. At least, this applies in Western societies though the converse may be seen in some developing countries where it is the more wealthy who are at increased risk of cardiovascular disease, presumably because they live long enough to develop it without succumbing to malnutrition and infectious diseases.

> *Lower socioeconomic class is strongly linked to higher blood pressures*

### The role of salt

Few topics in hypertension or perhaps any cardiovascular condition generate as much heated debate as the possible role of salt in the pathogenesis of hypertension. Most epidemiological data support the view that populations with high salt intakes have higher levels of blood pressure, with an approximately linear correlation.[13] This has obvious public health implications, since it is clear that most people in developed countries have salt intakes much higher than those needed for sodium and water homeostasis: a tendency reinforced by the sometimes extraordinarily high salt content of processed foods (although this may now be improving with increasing public awareness of the problem). Whether altering the salt intake of *individuals* will significantly modify their blood pressure, especially if it is already significantly raised, is a quite separate issue. The complexity of this question is further increased by recognition of the salt-sensitive phenotype already mentioned: it is therefore very likely that in some people salt-restriction will make a worthwhile difference, while in others the effect will be negligible.

> *In some people salt-restriction will make a worthwhile difference, while in others the effect will be negligible*

### Obesity

There can be no serious disagreement about the importance of weight and obesity, especially as regards diastolic blood pressure. It is much more difficult to determine why this is the case (Figure 9). Among the proposed mechanisms are hyperactivity of the sympathetic and renin-angiotensin systems, although these changes are not universally found and several alternatives are now being examined such as the involvement of the hypothalamic peptide orexin. Over the last 10–15 years it has become clear that there are several types of obesity, which, while they all may be associated with hypertension, have other important health implications:

> *There can be no serious disagreement about the importance of weight and obesity, especially as regards diastolic blood pressure*

- Generalized obesity[16] is a significant contributory factor in hypertension, probably by several mechanism, such as sleep apnoea (see below).
- Central or truncal obesity, with an increased waist:hip ratio and disproportionate accumulation of visceral, as opposed to subcutaneous, fat is associated with the metabolic syndrome[17,18] (also called syndrome X, very confusingly as there are lots of other syndrome Xs!). In these circumstances hypertension is part of a recognizable combination of metabolic abnormalities with very considerable implications for cardiovascular risk: this will be discussed in greater detail later.

*66Over the last 10–15 years it has become clear that there are several types of obesity 99*

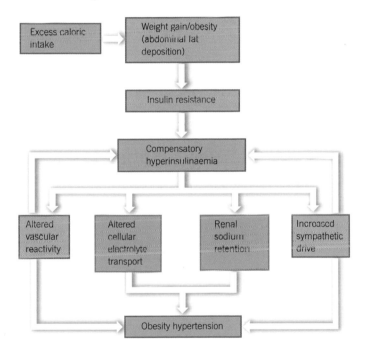

**Fig. 9 Possible pathogenic mechanisms of obesity hypertension.**

Reproduced with permission from Crawford et al. Cardiology. 2nd Edition. Mosby, 2004.

### Sympathetic overactivity

The *sympathetic nervous system* has already been mentioned on several occasions. There have been proposals that overactivity of this system is the fundamental problem in *all* hypertension. This is no longer considered to be very likely but there certainly appear to be circumstances where it is of critical importance. This is most notable in the early stages of hypertension where there may be increased cardiac output and resting pulse rate, but normal peripheral resistance. This pattern is quite frequent in young men with "borderline" hypertension

*66There have been proposals that sympathetic overactivity is the fundamental problem in all hypertension 99*

and they may demonstrate the white-coat effect particularly strongly. As we will discuss later, quite how to manage these individuals is one of the major clinical quandaries in hypertension.

The Folkow-Lever hypothesis of the pathogenesis of hypertension was outlined earlier. It is based on the concept that hypertension is initiated by "something" that produces vasoconstriction and that "something" could, at least in some individuals, be the sympathetic nervous system.

### Stress[19,20]

> *Most people perceive themselves to be stressed*

At some point many newly diagnosed hypertensives will ask health professionals (and themselves) whether the condition can be caused by stress, since most people perceive themselves to be stressed – and the perception means that they probably are. Among the possible answers is one that is certainly evasive and may be flippant: it all depends on what you mean by stress. This is true in at least two respects:

- Stress is not easy to quantify and the validity of relatively easily obtained parameters such as heart rate and plasma or urinary catecholamines is debatable, there being no "gold standard" measurement.

> *It is those at the lower rungs of corporate or political ladders that appear to be particularly stressed*

- In as far as stress is measurable, recent studies have contradicted widely held preconceptions. People at the top of hierarchies see themselves as under exceptional stress. This may be true in some circumstances, notably during crises, but under most conditions and at most times it is those at the lower rungs of corporate or political ladders that appear to be particularly stressed, probably reflecting their relatively limited ability to control their lives. Again this must impinge on the interactions of socioeconomic class and disease, including hypertension. Interesting light was shed on this by studies of Kenyan migrants from rural areas to Nairobi,[21] who showed significant blood pressure rises: a combination of socioeconomic stress and dietary change?

### Alcohol

> *In some cases those who actually did drink nothing at all had slightly higher blood pressures than moderate drinkers*

The relationship of alcohol consumption to blood pressure was the subject of a legendary survey of French army officers before the First World War, a pioneering study of its kind (Figure 10). It found that heavy drinkers had significantly raised blood pressure – though to put this in context those who drank less than two bottles of wine a day were essentially considered to be teetotal! Later studies on lower average consumption levels have confirmed this finding, with the proviso that in some cases those who actually did drink nothing at all had slightly higher blood pressures than moderate drinkers. Possible

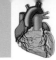

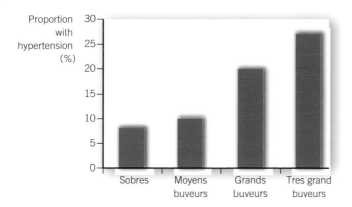

**Fig. 10 Hypertension and alcohol** – C. Lian, French army physician, 1915.

Definitions:

| | |
|---|---|
| Sobres | < 1 litre wine/day |
| Moyens buveurs | 1–1.5 litres wine/day |
| Grands buveurs | 2–2.5 litres wine/day |
| Tres grand buveurs | ≥ 3 litres wine/day + 4–6 aperitifs |

mechanisms for this include weight gain due to the considerable calorie equivalence of alcohol and of the non-alcohol content of some drinks especially beer; increased sympathetic activity; and a cushingoid syndrome with increased cortisol secretion. Binge drinkers are at particular risk of stroke associated with acute increases in blood pressure, and dramatic rises in blood pressure can also occur during withdrawal from alcohol in physically dependent alcoholic subjects.

> **Binge drinkers are at particular risk of stroke associated with acute increases in blood pressure**

### A special case: isolated systolic hypertension

It has already been pointed out that in diastolic, or usually systolo-diastolic, hypertension the final common pathway is increased peripheral resistance. This implies alterations in small arteries, arterioles and capillaries. In isolated systolic hypertension (ISH)[7] this does not appear to be the case: the problem is in the larger arteries. These become progressively more rigid and inelastic and therefore reflect and amplify the pulse wave (this is of course a great oversimplification of an extremely complex problem in fluid dynamics). Therefore ISH reflects the ageing process itself as it affects the arterial tree. Perhaps surprisingly, the different pathophysiologies of the two types of hypertension make little difference to the choice of treatments for the two conditions.

> **ISH reflects the ageing process itself as it affects the arterial tree**

## Secondary hypertension: the more common rarities

Since we are dealing with a small minority of the hypertensive population even the most common of these conditions will present only occasionally among those seen by primary or even secondary care physicians. This does not mean that their detection is irrelevant: sometimes it is of great importance even if it does not immediately improve the management of the blood pressure as such. The kidney is prominent as a cause of secondary hypertension, indeed it may be central to primary hypertension. The kidney may be a culprit in but also a victim of hypertension, and sometimes both simultaneously.

> *" The kidney is prominent as a cause of secondary hypertension "*

### Renal parenchymal disease

Most patients with severe or even moderate uncorrected renal failure are hypertensive and they may have extremely high blood pressure that is very refractory to treatment. This will occur regardless of the underlying cause of the disease. The main reason for this is almost certainly related to extracellular volume expansion with secondary neurohumoral changes that reinforce the process. There is also a high incidence of hypertension in transplant patients, partly due to their drug therapies, and in those on dialysis, though they are likely to have less severe problems than those without adequate treatment. Most chronic renal disease is not curable and even when it is there is no certainty that the hypertension will be reversible.

> *" Most chronic renal disease is not curable "*

### Renovascular disease[22,23]

This is a much more difficult and contentious area in terms of diagnosis and management. Renovascular disease implies that there is a stenosis, or several lesions, affecting the arterial supply to one or both kidneys (Figure 11). This corresponds with animal models of hypertension with respect to the stimulation of renin release. The

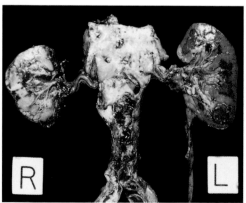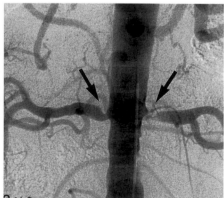

**Fig. 11 Bilateral renovascular disease with severe atheromatous disease (left).** The individual had accelerated hypertension. Reproduced with kind permission from Graham A MacGregor. **Renal artery lesions (right).** Aortogram from a patient with moderate hypertension and normal renal function. Reproduced with permission from Hallett et al. Comprehensive vascular and endovascular surgery. Mosby, 2004.

chronic and sometimes progressive ischaemia can lead to progressive renal impairment and even loss of the kidney, which may occur catastrophically because of arterial thrombosis. Renal artery stenosis may however present as hypertension or as heart failure, occurring chronically or as an acute emergency, or occasionally with a mixed clinical picture. There are two main subsets of the population that are likely to suffer from this condition, or rather conditions. They are:

- young people, typically women in their 20s
- individuals over the age of 50 years, more commonly men.

The pathology is quite different in these two groups. Typically, younger people are suffering from a condition of unknown aetiology called fibromuscular hyperplasia, which gradually encroaches on the lumen, while in the older patient the lesion is usually an atheromatous plaque or plaques. The approaches to diagnosis will be discussed later and present perhaps unexpected complexities but the crucial question is: to what extent does correction of the stenosis correlate with improvement or even cure of the hypertension? The answer is on the whole disappointing for the older patient though generally much more positive for the younger patient with fibromuscular stenosis.

*"The chronic and sometimes progressive ischaemia can lead to progressive renal impairment and even loss of the kidney"*

### Primary hyperaldosteronism: Conn's syndrome[24]

For many years after its discovery Conn's syndrome was reputed to be an extremely rare condition associated with mild to moderate hypertension: neither of these perceptions is quite correct. In fact, many clinicians now believe that the incidence of Conn's syndrome in hypertensive populations approaches that of renal disease, so that it is one of the most important causes of secondary hypertension although one that has almost certainly been underdiagnosed (Figure 12).

*"Conn's syndrome is one of the most important causes of secondary hypertension"*

| Clinical features of primary aldosteronism |
| --- |
| • Muscle weakness |
| • Cramps and tetany |
| • Polyuria |
| • Low serum $K^+$ |
| • High normal or high serum $Na^+$ |
| • High serum $HCO_3^-$ |

Fig. 12 Clinical features of primary hyperaldosteronism.

Hypokalaemia is of course an important clue: it is clear that some patients with this syndrome have normal plasma levels of potassium, though hypokalaemia may become manifest if the patients are treated with even very low doses of diuretics such as thiazides. In addition, severe and even malignant hypertension certainly occurs in these

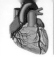
patients and their blood pressure may not be at all easy to control. The source of excess aldosterone may be bilateral adrenal hyperplasia or a unilateral adenoma and the differentiation between these two possibilities may alter approaches to therapy, although to a lesser extent than formerly. Many patients, even with unilateral adenomas, refuse surgery and prefer indefinite medical treatment. This is based, logically enough, on the specific aldosterone receptor antagonist spironolactone, which should reduce blood pressure and correct the hypokalaemia, though usually additional drugs are needed, such as the potassium-sparing diuretic amiloride and the calcium-channel blocker amlodipine.

## Secondary hypertension: rarer rarities
### Phaeochromocytoma[25]

This is a very rare but highly dramatic and also very dangerous form of hypertension. Typically, but by no means invariably, the hypertension follows an episodic pattern in keeping with releases of catecholamines from the chromaffin cell tumours. These tumours are most often found in the adrenal glands (Figures 13 and 14) but can arise from any collection

**Fig. 13  Symptoms and signs of phaeochromocytoma.**

Reproduced with permission from Swales JD and De Bono DP. Slide Atlas of Cardiovascular Risk Factors. London: Elsevier, 1993.

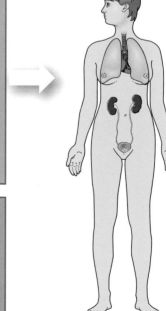

- Paroxysmal hypertension
- Headache
- Pallor/flush
- Anxiety
- Thyroid swelling
- Chest pain
- Palpitation
- Tachycardia
- Nausea/vomiting
- Glycosuria
- Sweating
- Tremor
- Weakness

Tests for localization
- Venous catheter
- CT scan
- Arteriogram
- MIBG radioactive localization
- VMA/metanephrine/
  free metanephrine (urine)
- Epinephrine/
  norepinephrine (blood)

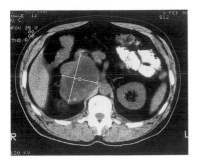 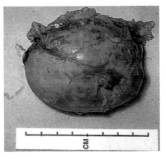

**Fig. 14**
**Phaeochromocytoma.**
CT scan of tumour *in situ* (left). Surgically excised tumour (right).

Reproduced with permission from MacGregor GA. Diagnostic picture tests in hypertension. London: Elsevier Ltd, 1996.

of sympathetic nerve cells, for instance adjacent to the bladder or at the aortic bifurcation. The tumour may form part of the familial multiple endocrine adenomata syndromes. The surges in blood pressure may be dangerously high and are characteristically accompanied by anxiety, pallor and sweating. Since the predominant catecholamine is noradrenaline in the great majority (about 90%) of cases, palpitations are not rapid but may be abnormally slow due to reflex bradycardia secondary to intense vasoconstriction. These tumours are especially dangerous during surgery and pregnancy but the blood pressure peaks can occur unpredictably at any time. There is also the danger of malignant, sarcomatous transformation in the tumours so that there is no question that they should be removed if at all possible. Hypertension will certainly be alleviated and may disappear altogether. Pending surgery, or if surgery is refused by the patient or is for some reason not feasible, treatment is focused on complete alpha-adrenoceptor blockade, usually with the irreversible antagonist phenoxybenzamine. It is absolutely vital not to give these patients beta-blockers unless total alpha-blockade is established, otherwise one might see unopposed vasoconstriction occurring, with potentially disastrous increases in blood pressure.

> **❝There is no question that phaeochromo-cytoma should be removed if at all possible ❞**

### Cushing's syndrome

This condition may arise from unilateral adrenal adenomas, bilateral adrenal hyperplasia, or as an adrenal response to excessive pituitary secretion of ACTH. Given the other components of the syndrome, hypertension may not be a presenting feature. As with Conn's syndrome, volume expansion is likely to be a major contributory mechanism and it is likely that hypokalaemia will be found. Primary treatment of the syndrome will almost certainly reduce blood pressure levels but may not normalize them.

> **❝Primary treatment of the syndrome will almost certainly reduce blood pressure levels but may not normalize them ❞**

### Hyperparathyroidism

A less well known and rather puzzling cause, or apparent cause, of hypertension. At least 50% of patients with this condition are hypertensive. Parathormone is not a vasoconstrictor and severity of hypertension does not correlate well with serum levels of either calcium or parathormone. One factor may be increasing arterial stiffness perhaps associated with calcium deposition in the vessel wall. Once again, parathyroidectomy and normalization of serum calcium levels does not by any means guarantee abolition of the hypertension.

> ❝ *Coarctation of the aorta is usually detected in childhood but may not present until well into adult life* ❞

### Coarctation of the aorta

This rare form of hypertension is usually detected in childhood but may not present until well into adult life, especially if the narrowing is relatively mild (Figures 15–17). On the other hand, later surgery is less likely to produce a definitive cure of the hypertension. Part of the

**Fig. 15 Coarctation of the aorta (right). Normal tricuspid aortic valve (left).** Reproduced with permission from Fowler. Diagnosis in color: Physical signs in cardiology. Mosby, 1999.

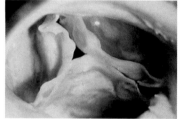
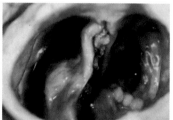

**Fig. 16 Direct recording of brachial and femoral blood pressures in a patient with aortic coarctation.** Note that not only is the peak femoral systolic pressure lower than the brachial pressure but also that the femoral pulse is delayed. Reproduced with permission from Fowler. Diagnosis in color: Physical signs in cardiology. Mosby, 1999.

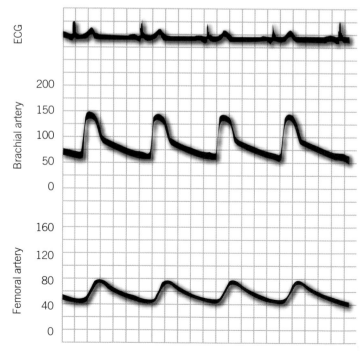

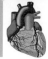

| Signs and symptoms of coarctation |
| --- |
| • Systolic murmur over back and collaterals |
| • Large left ventricle |
| • Rib notches (on X-ray) |
| • Claudication |
| • Arterial neck pulsation |
| • Radial/femoral delay |
| • Cold feet |

**Fig. 17 Clinical signs and symptoms of aortic coarctation.** Reproduced with permission from Slide Atlas of Cardiovascular Risk Factors. Elsevier.

mechanism of the raised blood pressure may relate to renal ischaemia leading to activation of the renin-angiotensin system.

### Obstructive sleep apnoea[26]

The existence of this syndrome has gained increased recognition and with this has come the realization that it has important cardiovascular implications, especially hypertension. Although the stereotyped patient is the middle-aged overweight male, and this does represent the largest single group, it can affect any individual. One estimate suggests that as many as one in 15 adults may have moderate to severe sleep apnoea. Several lines of evidence support the link between sleep apnoea and hypertension: though the mechanism is uncertain it is likely to involve increased sympathetic activation. Polysomnography is the definitive diagnostic approach together with oximetry, though of course the history particularly from the patient's partner is often crucial. The lack of nocturnal dipping in 24-hour blood pressure monitoring is also suggestive. Attempts should be made to correct the apnoea, with continuous positive airway pressure (CPAP) being the most effective option. There is as yet no reliable outcome data, but it is unlikely that correction of the apnoea will by itself normalize the blood pressure.

*"One in 15 adults may have moderate to severe sleep apnoea"*

### The metabolic syndrome[17,18]

Although it is important that the above-listed conditions are not missed, no one is under any illusion that they have major significance at a population level. The metabolic syndrome (now much the most widely accepted term) is of a different order of importance and is particularly significant among middle-aged men and in some ethnic groups. It is of course simplistic to think of it primarily as a cause of hypertension. Raised blood pressure is only one element in an aggregate of clinical problems (Figure 18) that greatly increase the risk of cardiovascular disease. Insulin resistance, that is to say the failure of peripheral tissues to respond to circulating insulin is at the core of the

*"Raised blood pressure is only one element in an aggregate of clinical problems"*

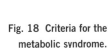

**Fig. 18 Criteria for the metabolic syndrome.**

| **Usually includes three of the following:** |
| --- |
| • Raised fasting blood glucose* |
| • Dyslipidaemia (low HDL cholesterol, raised triglycerides) |
| • Abdominal obesity (usually defined as waist circumference >102 cm for men, >88 cm for women) |
| • Raised blood pressure* |
| *Thresholds vary: 5.6–6.1 mmol/l for glucose; systolic 130–140 mmHg for blood pressure |

syndrome. This finding, which is not uniform in all tissues, in turn leads to glucose intolerance and elevated glucose levels after a carbohydrate load. The precise sequence of events in the metabolic syndrome is the subject of intense debate and research, and increasingly the role of visceral fat is considered crucially important, possibly with the release of inflammatory cytokines from central adipose tissue: sympathetic nervous system overactivity may also play a part. It is doubtful whether the metabolic syndrome is "curable" in the usual sense of the word but it can certainly be improved. However, lowering blood pressure is not in itself effective in this respect: some antihypertensive drugs may improve glucose tolerance (possibly ACE inhibitors and angiotensin II receptor antagonists) while others may make it worse (probably thiazide diuretics and the conventional beta-blockers). Whether this actually alters clinical outcomes one way or the other is another source of controversy: one would expect that it would, but that is no guarantee that it does!

> *It is doubtful whether the metabolic syndrome is "curable" in the usual sense of the word but it can certainly be improved*

### Hypertension in different ethnic groups[27]

It must be clear from the discussion to date that the condition known as hypertension is very heterogeneous. Hardly surprisingly, it is possible to detect the heterogeneity that is associated with different ethnic groups. Two examples are reasonably well characterized:

> *The metabolic syndrome is particularly common among men of South Asian origin*

- The metabolic syndrome is particularly common among men of South Asian origin, especially among those living in Western societies. The reasons for this are still not well understood but these individuals are unquestionably at high risk of premature coronary heart disease.
- Black populations in the UK, USA and the Caribbean have higher rates of hypertension than other ethnic groups. It is also higher than the incidence in West Africa, the original home from which these populations were involuntary migrants. However, those who

move into other environments from West Africa also show an increased incidence of hypertension. Hypertension in this population has many characteristic features including:

- very low or even undetectable levels of circulating renin
- considerable sensitivity to salt
- higher prevalence of left ventricular hypertrophy and renal damage.

Related to the first two of these, black hypertensives have different sensitivities to some of the most commonly used antihypertensive agents.

> **"Black hypertensives have different sensitivities to some of the most commonly used antihypertensive agents"**

## Drug-induced hypertension

Doctors are an important cause of hypertension. Many drugs, both prescribed and otherwise, can cause acute or chronic rises in blood pressure, again emphasizing the importance of an accurate drug history in patient assessment. Many of these drugs are in very wide usage, as this section will show. Of course, non-prescribed drugs, even "natural" ones, may be equally hazardous.

### Corticosteroids

Iatrogenic Cushing's syndrome can be associated with hypertension in the same way as the spontaneous disease. This effect is dose dependent and not everyone is affected even at high doses of systemic steroids: it is also possible that a few patients treated with high-potency steroids for skin disease may absorb enough to produce hypertension. Certainly monitoring of blood pressure is essential in all patients receiving steroids systemically.

> **"A few patients treated with high-potency steroids for skin disease may absorb enough to produce hypertension"**

### Oral contraceptive pill and hormone replacement therapy[28]

Although most women taking the combined oral contraceptive (COC) pill show small rises in blood pressure a minority, about 5%, have a significant increase in pressure and a very small number develop malignant or accelerated hypertension. There is research in progress to examine a possible link between the exaggerated hypertensive response and a history of migraine. It is thought that it is the oestrogenic component of the COC that is responsible for the blood pressure effects, which are dose related. It seems that progestogen-only pills lack this adverse effect, which is thought to be due to sodium retention and activation of the renin-angiotensin system.

By contrast, women taking hormone replacement therapy (HRT) seem not to be at enhanced risk of hypertension. This discrepancy may reflect the fact that the oestrogens used in the two situations are completely different.

> **"It is thought that it is the oestrogenic component of the COC that is responsible for the blood pressure effects"**

27

### Non-steroidal anti-inflammatory drugs (NSAIDs)

These are among the most commonly prescribed and self-administered drugs in the world. Unfortunately the group most likely to suffer serious adverse effects, the elderly, are also those most likely to take the drugs. NSAIDs increase sodium and water retention and reduce overall renal function in many individuals.[29] They may directly cause hypertension in some susceptible individuals, though this appears to be rare. More importantly, they can counteract the antihypertensive effects of several classes of drugs, including thiazides and ACE inhibitors but probably not calcium-channel blockers. This provides an additional reason, beyond gastrointestinal toxicity, for limiting the long-term use of these drugs. Despite earlier expectations, it is now almost certain that the new COX-2 selective drugs are as likely to cause renal and hypertensive adverse effects as the older non-selective agents.[30] In fact, it has been suggested that they may actually increase cardiovascular risk in comparison with conventional NSAIDs. The rationale for this is the fact that COX-2 inhibitors reduce endothelial prostacyclin synthesis, which is partly COX-2 mediated, but do not affect platelet activation, since only COX-1 is present in the platelet. At present there is no convincing evidence of enhanced risk, though there may prove to be significant differences between drugs in this class and some may be safer than others.

> 66 *NSAIDs can counteract the antihypertensive effects of several classes of drugs* 99

### Cyclosporin and tacrolimus[31]

Cyclosporin is nephrotoxic but it is thought that this does not wholly explain its effect on blood pressure, which may include direct effects on small blood vessels. At least 25% of treated individuals become hypertensive but in some series almost every patient was affected. Since in many cases drug withdrawal is not feasible this is an unwelcome example of the adverse effects of one drug requiring treatment with other drugs, in this case usually calcium-channel blockers. It was hoped that the newer immunosuppressant tacrolimus would have a lower incidence of renal and blood pressure problems and this appears to be the case.

> 66 *In many cases drug withdrawal is not feasible* 99

### Erythropoietin[32]

This vitally important treatment for the anaemia of end-stage renal disease causes hypertension in about a third of treated patients, in a small minority leading to dangerously high blood pressure levels. Relatively rapid increases in haematocrit may be relevant but other factors must also be involved. Needless to say, the rise in blood pressure, unless dangerously high, is not an indication for stopping the drug, although it might make difficult hypertension even harder to manage.

### Sympathomimetic drugs

Drugs of this class (ephedrine, pseudoephedrine and phenyl-propanolamine) are widely bought over the counter as decongestant cold remedies and, though certainly unlicensed for this indication, as slimming aids often at high doses. Since they can cause generalized vasoconstriction it is hardly surprising that they can cause hypertension and that this may be severe. Phenylpropanolamine has now been withdrawn in most countries after numerous case reports of severe hypertension associated with strokes. Some ephedrine containing preparations have also been withdrawn recently in the USA.

> **"Phenylpropanol-amine has now been withdrawn in most countries after numerous case reports of severe hypertension associated with strokes"**

### Liquorice

Liquorice contains carbenoxolone, a steroid that was used as an anti-ulcer agent before the introduction of $H_2$ antagonists. In quite modest quantities this compound can induce a primary hyperaldosteronism-like clinical picture with hypertension and hypokalaemia. This is actually an indirect effect, caused by inhibition of an enzyme that protects mineralocorticoid receptors from inappropriate activation. The aldosterone receptor antagonist spironolactone effectively antagonizes the pressor activity of liquorice/carbenoxolone.

### Recreational drugs

Many of these, legal or otherwise, have the potential to promote or worsen hypertension. This will be discussed briefly.

**Nicotine,** when smoked but apparently not in the form of transdermal patches, acutely increases blood pressure. Tolerance does not develop to this response, which is thought to be mediated by a central effect on sympathetic drive. However, the pressor response is transient and there is no clear link between smoking and sustained hypertension: there have even been suggestions of a negative correlation, though this rather surprising and questionable observation hardly cancels the many other reasons for advising people to stop smoking!

> **"There is no clear link between smoking and sustained hypertension"**

**Caffeine,** on the other hand, appears to cause both transient and persistent elevations in blood pressure and this influences basal blood pressure in both normotensive and hypertensive individuals. The importance of this in patients with established hypertension is a matter of debate; as usual moderation (less than four cups of coffee a day, for instance) seems a reasonable approach, though some patients make the decision to drink only decaffeinated beverages.

*Cocaine and amphetamines* cause paroxysmal rather than sustained increases in blood pressure. However, these may be severe enough to cause cerebral haemorrhage.

*Alcohol* is discussed elsewhere, and it is just worth noting here that it can be a contributor to raised blood pressure by its action on the sympathetic nervous system and also as a major source of calories in some overweight and obese individuals (though the latter point has recently been questioned by some researchers in the Czech Republic!).

*Khat* is a plant grown in the hills of Somalia, Ethiopia, Eritrea and the Yemen. It is legally and widely available in the UK and used regularly by many men from these communities. Its active ingredient, cathinone, is a powerful sympathomimetic and can cause severe paroxysmal and sustained increases in blood pressure.[34]

## Consequences of hypertension

Although the causes of hypertension are surrounded by controversy and uncertainty, we do have a better understanding of the consequences of raised arterial blood pressure. That of course is the reason we are interested in this condition as clinicians, not because of obsessions about achieving normal readings when we measure blood pressure. The principal organs damaged by high blood pressure are:

- the heart
- the kidney
- the brain
- large and small blood vessels.

### Cardiac effects of hypertension

For most people the idea that the heart has to work harder in the presence of hypertension seems right intuitively, and of course it is true. The consequences of this are more complex however than appear to be the case.

*The idea that the heart has to work harder in the presence of hypertension seems right intuitively*

#### Left ventricular hypertrophy (Figure 19 and 20)

The best-known and most readily understandable result of sustained hypertension. It entails increased muscle mass and wall thickness, and it is now clear that there is also a variable component of fibrosis. This should not obscure the fact that the hypertrophic response is mediated by more than just increased resistance and the mechanical consequences that follow. The role of the renin-angiotensin-aldosterone system has attracted particular attention recently and it is likely that endothelin is also involved, although peptide itself, this

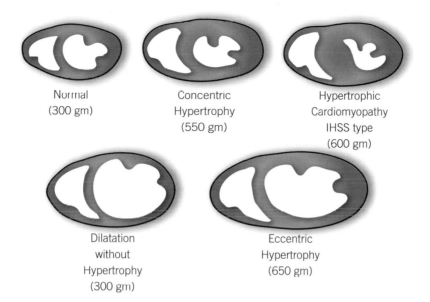

| Normal<br>(300 gm) | Concentric<br>Hypertrophy<br>(550 gm) | Hypertrophic<br>Cardiomyopathy<br>IHSS type<br>(600 gm) |
|---|---|---|

| Dilatation<br>without<br>Hypertrophy<br>(300 gm) | Eccentric<br>Hypertrophy<br>(650 gm) |
|---|---|

clearly interacts with the renin system. There has been very lively debate about the relative efficacy of different antihypertensive drugs and a consensus has now been reached that ACE inhibitors and angiotensin II receptor antagonists are more effective than beta-blockers and possibly than other agents in the partial reversal of left ventricular hypertrophy.[34,35] As with the vascular changes in hypertension the left ventricle can respond by either hypertrophy or

**Fig. 19 Left ventricular hypertrophy.** Typical figures for left ventricular masses are indicated, much higher figures are sometimes seen.

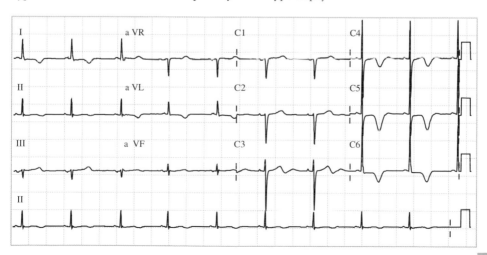

**Fig. 20 Left ventricular hypertrophy – 12 lead ECG.** Note typical deep S waves in C(V)2 and tall R wave in C(V)5

remodelling though some form of hypertrophy is usual. On theoretical grounds pressure overload alone should lead to concentric hypertrophy but in fact the eccentric pattern is more common. Some investigators believe that concentric hypertrophy has more serious implications than other patterns, but this is far from a unanimous view.

Left ventricular hypertrophy is much more than an indicator that hypertension has been and is present.[36] The presence of hypertrophy is associated with at least a doubling of the risk of cardiovascular mortality and morbidity. There are three main reasons for this:

- There is increased likelihood of serious ventricular dysrhythmias, because of altered electrical connections between hypertrophied cardiac myocytes and also because of disruption of intraventricular conduction pathways by fibrosis.
- The circulatory reserve within the myocardium may not keep pace with the increasing demands of the hypertrophied tissue, leading to increasing ischaemia, which in turn may be a contributory factor for heart failure.
- The development of heart failure. Hypertension is the second most common cause of heart failure in the UK, after ischaemic heart disease with which it may often co-exist. Diastolic dysfunction is an early feature of established hypertension and reflects increasing stiffness of the hypertrophied and fibrotic ventricle. To some extent this also occurs as a part of ageing without hypertension but raised blood pressure very much exaggerates the process. In the majority of hypertensive patients who develop clinical heart failure it is characterized by systolic dysfunction, with a reduced ejection fraction. However, in about 40% of patients the primary abnormality is diastolic, with largely preserved systolic function. The recognition of this syndrome is fairly recent and its implications for treatment are still uncertain: however, it is very important to note that the diagnosis of heart failure cannot be excluded even when the ejection fraction is unremarkable.

*" The presence of hypertrophy is associated with at least a doubling of the risk of cardiovascular mortality and morbidity "*

*" Hypertension is the second most common cause of heart failure in the UK "*

## Hypertension and the kidney (Figure 21)

As already mentioned, the kidney is very much implicated as a cause of hypertension but is also one of the organs most likely to be damaged by it. It is generally believed that, before the advent of effective antihypertensive treatment, most patients with severe disease died of renal failure. Today cardiovascular and cerebrovascular complications are much more important as causes of death and morbidity. Nonetheless, most experts consider that the effects of poorly controlled hypertension on the kidneys are of major importance, especially in the presence of diabetes. The characteristic renal lesion in hypertensive

*" Before the advent of effective antihypertensive treatment, most patients with severe disease died of renal failure "*

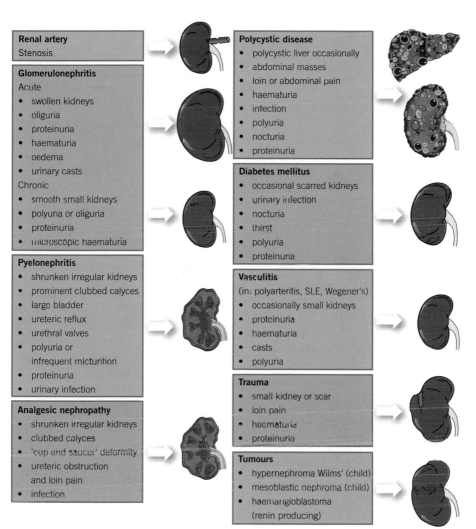

**Renal artery**
Stenosis

**Glomerulonephritis**
Acute
- swollen kidneys
- oliguria
- proteinuria
- haematuria
- oedema
- urinary casts
Chronic
- smooth small kidneys
- polyuria or oliguria
- proteinuria
- microscopic haematuria

**Pyelonephritis**
- shrunken irregular kidneys
- prominent clubbed calyces
- large bladder
- ureteric reflux
- urethral valves
- polyuria or
  infrequent micturition
- proteinuria
- urinary infection

**Analgesic nephropathy**
- shrunken irregular kidneys
- clubbed calyces
- 'cup and saucer' deformity
- ureteric obstruction
  and loin pain
- infection

**Polycystic disease**
- polycystic liver occasionally
- abdominal masses
- loin or abdominal pain
- haematuria
- infection
- polyuria
- nocturia
- proteinuria

**Diabetes mellitus**
- occasional scarred kidneys
- urinary infection
- nocturia
- thirst
- polyuria
- proteinuria

**Vasculitis**
(in: polyarteritis, SLE, Wegener's)
- occasionally small kidneys
- proteinuria
- haematuria
- casts
- polyuria

**Trauma**
- small kidney or scar
- loin pain
- haematuria
- proteinuria

**Tumours**
- hypernephroma Wilms' (child)
- mesoblastic nephroma (child)
- haemangioblastoma
  (renin producing)

renal damage is nephrosclerosis, involving the afferent arterioles. Some writers have questioned the association of renal damage and hypertension, holding the view that apparent hypertensive injury reflects only the aggravation of pre-existing renal disease, which in turn may be a contributory factor in the development of hypertension. Like so many other issues relating to the kidneys and blood pressure this remains in some doubt. In any case, initially micro- and later macro-albuminuria (see below) reflect renal damage and predict deteriorating renal function and the prospective risk of cardiovascular complications.

**Fig. 21 Renal disorders associated with hypertension.** Reproduced with permission from Swales JD and De Bono DP. Slide Atlas of Cardiovascular Risk Factors. London: Elsevier, 1993.

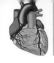

As previously noted, renal damage is apparently more common in black hypertensives than in other groups at comparable levels of blood pressure.

## Hypertension and the brain

> 66 *Stroke is the best known and most feared complication of hypertension* 99

Stroke is the best known and most feared complication of hypertension. Yet many of the general perceptions of this often lethal or disabling event are mistaken. First, the intuitive view is that most strokes are "burst" blood vessels. In fact about 5% of strokes in hypertensive patients are due to subarachnoid haemorrhage, another 5–15% are intracerebral haemorrhages (Figure 22) but the remaining

**Fig. 22 Intracerebral haematoma.** High blood pressure is believed to be primarily responsible for about half of all cases. Reproduced with permission from Clinical Atlas of Cerebrovascular Disorders edited by Marc Fisher. Wolfe Publishing, 1994.

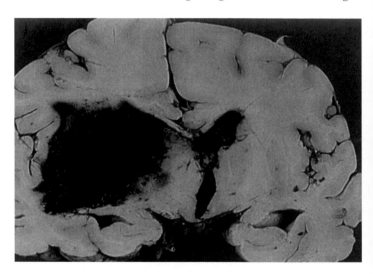

80% are thrombotic or thromboembolic involving vessels of any size from the common carotid to intracerebral arterioles. Mural plaque in the carotids is a common source of small emboli, such as those causing amaurosis fugax. The reasons for small vessel thrombosis are less easy to delineate but the concept of a prothrombotic state associated with hypertension[37] has been discussed and may be due, at least in part, to endothelial dysfunction, though there are also changes in circulating coagulation and fibrinolytic factors.

> 66 *About half of the strokes in treated hypertensives occur when the blood pressure is normal by any criteria* 99

Second, it is widely believed that strokes occur when the blood pressure is very high. It is true that the higher the pressure the higher the risk, particularly if the rise in pressure is rapid as in the "morning surge". However, the mean pressure at which strokes occur is only 150/90mmHg, only 10mmHg above current treatment targets. Nevertheless, about half of the strokes in treated hypertensives occur when the blood pressure is normal by any criteria, indicating either that antihypertensive therapy does not necessarily correct the abnormalities of the untreated condition, or that current criteria of normality are not stringent enough, or very likely both.

However, we need to extend our thinking about the effects of hypertension on the brain beyond the consideration of stroke. Hypertension is almost certainly associated with accelerated cognitive decline even without detectable strokes (Figure 23).[39] Some clinical

***"Hypertension is almost certainly associated with accelerated cognitive decline even without detectable strokes "***

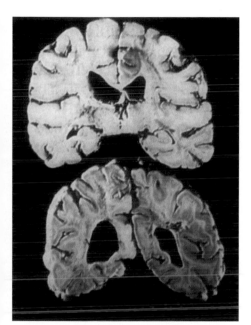

**Fig. 23  Brain lesions in Binswanger's disease.**
Hypertension is a known risk factor for this chronic cerebrovascular disease, which is a form of senile dementia. Note the extensive white-matter lesions and dilated ventricles.

Reproduced with permission from Clinical Atlas of Cerebrovascular Disorders edited by Marc Fisher. Wolfe Publishing, 1994.

trials have suggested that effective blood pressure control may prevent or at least modify this process but this has not been seen in other trials: however, inhibition of angiotensin II receptors may be particularly useful.[40] More studies are needed to reach a definitive conclusion but in practical terms the case for good control of blood pressure can only be further strengthened even if there is no definitive proof of a link.

One important related issue concerns the risks of aspirin in hypertensive patients. It is of course the case that aspirin carries haemorrhagic risk even at the lowest dose. But, specifically, patients with uncontrolled hypertension taking aspirin are at increased risk of intracerebral haemorrhage. It is not clear what level of control should be considered acceptable: there are no real prospective data and decisions are therefore rather arbitrary. It has been proposed that 150/90mmHg might serve as a realistic cut-off point.

***"Patients with uncontrolled hypertension taking aspirin are at increased risk of intracerebral haemorrhage "***

## Hypertension and arteries

The common feature in all the consequences of hypertension described in this section is, of course, the damage to blood vessels. This takes several forms depending on the size and site of the artery:

- Aorta hypertension is a factor, often the major one, in the pathogenesis of acute dissection, one of the real hypertensive emergencies (Figure 24). Presumably there is direct damage from the peak of the pulse wave as well as accelerated atherosclerosis: it is not clear how important atherosclerosis is. Hypertension is commonly listed as a risk factor for abdominal aortic aneurysm but in fact the association is not strong and incidence of aortic aneurysm in hypertensive patients is well under 10%, though it approaches this level in patients with severe systolic hypertension (around 200mmHg).

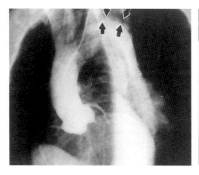 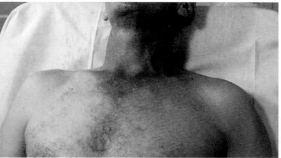

**Fig. 24 Dissecting aortic aneurysm.**
Aortogram (left) with arrows indicating the site of compression of the left innominate vein by the dissecting aneurysm. Distention of the left external jugular vein (right) as a result of compression of the left innominate vein.
Reproduced with permission from Fowler. Diagnosis in color: Physical signs in cardiology. Mosby, 1999.

- In the carotids increased intima-media thickness is an early indicator of atherosclerosis and may be a prognostic marker for cardiovascular disease. Hypertension accelerates these changes but is not considered to be a prime cause. This is the general view for the role of hypertension in medium-sized arteries: as a promoter of atherosclerosis but not in itself the primary cause. Similar considerations apply to peripheral vascular disease affecting the lower limbs.

- The same argument applies to the coronary arteries. It is interesting to note the interaction with other potential risk factors. Until recently coronary disease was rare in Japan, where hypertension was frequent and often severe, but cholesterol levels were low. With an increasingly Western lifestyle but better control of blood pressure the incidence of stroke has declined, approaching Western levels but that of ischaemic heart disease is increasing. It is still well below that of the UK however!

- The small arteries and arterioles have already been discussed in the context of the pathogenesis of hypertension. These changes can be

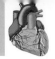

regarded as adaptive responses to increased blood pressure, though they do themselves help to maintain that increase. In extreme circumstances the vessel is irreversibly damaged. This condition, fibrinoid necrosis, is now very rarely seen since malignant hypertension is itself uncommon. For many years it was regarded as a common vascular lesion. The retina is of course the one site where these vessels can be directly examined (Figure 25).

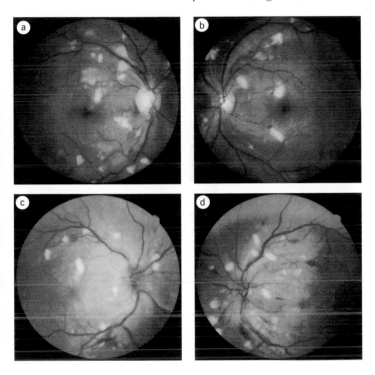

**Fig. 25  Keith-Wagener Grades III and IV hypertensive retinopathy.** (a, b) Grade III retinopathy showing attenuated arterioles and venous dilatation. Multiple widespread cotton-wool spots suggesting ischaemic fundi. (c, d) Grade IV retinopathy showing bilateral optic disc swelling (papilloedema) and widespread cotton-wool spots, macula stars and flame-shaped haemorrhages with attenuated arterioles.

Reproduced with permission from Lip et al. Fundal changes in malignant hypertension. J Hum Hypertens 1997;11:395–6. © 1997 Stockton Press.

## Diagnosing and assessing hypertension (Figure 26)

Having established the criteria for hypertension, as discussed earlier, diagnosis is surely simplicity itself. The response to that must be: if only! The principles are naturally the same as for any other clinical condition or syndrome, but, as usual, one needs to adapt to the specific circumstances. This will be followed through the usual stages, assuming the simplest scenario (if there is one); a middle-aged man or woman who is asymptomatic and comes for a routine check-up. Their blood pressure is persistently found to be 160/100mmHg, the measurement itself being discussed later. How do we adapt the "usual processes" to this condition?

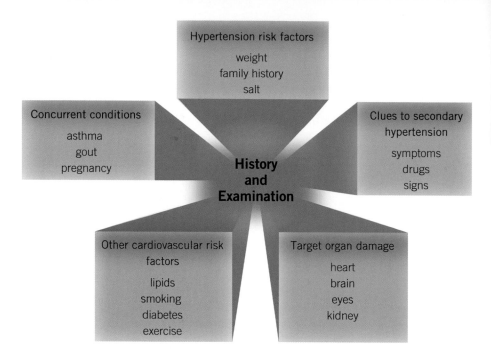

Fig. 26 History taking and examinations for hypertension.

### Clinical history (Figure 27)

Hypertension is, very largely, an asymptomatic condition until and unless it is very severe. Headache although often associated with hypertension in many people's minds, has no particular connection with mild to moderate hypertension, however:

1. Severe hypertension is often, but not always, associated with headache.
2. Some treated hypertensive individuals do experience headaches when their blood pressure rises above its usual, now reduced, level.
3. Many researchers believe that migraine is more common in hypertensive patients, and *vice versa*.

Chest pain, shortness of breath and palpitations may be symptoms of cardiac dysfunction, more often a consequence of ischaemic heart disease than of high blood pressure as such, but as already noted hypertension is itself a factor in the development of coronary artery disease.

Claudication and visual and other neurological symptoms may similarly reflect non-coronary arterial disease.

Polyuria and polydipsia may indicate concomitant diabetes, or renal dysfunction.

*" Hypertension is, very largely, an asymptomatic condition until and unless it is very severe "*

Morning headache
Seizures
Cerebral oedema
Visual disturbances and
   retinopathy papilloedema
Stroke (droop mouth,
   slurred speech, paresis)

**Fig. 27 Symptoms and signs associated with hypertension.** Reproduced with permission from Swales JD and De Bono DP. Slide Atlas of Cardiovascular Risk Factors. London: Elsevier, 1993.

Polyuria
Nocturia
Haematuria
Proteinuria
Dysuria

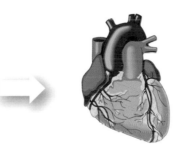

Right ventricular failure
   (third heart sound)
Left ventricular failure
   (fourth heart sound)
Gallop failure (left and right)
Angina pectoris
Myocardial infarction
Orthopnoea
Pulmonary oedema
Dyspnoea
Shortness of breath (on effort)
Intermittent claudication
Ankle oedema
Cold blue toes
Prominent pulsatile neck veins
Hepatomegaly (cardiac failure)
Systolic murmur

*66A history of hypertension or pre-eclampsia during pregnancy makes the subsequent development of essential hypertension much more likely 99*

Absent pulses
Unequal pulses

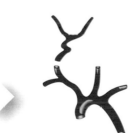

## Past medical history

Any indication of previous or current renal disease is of course very important, but this too may be asymptomatic for much of its clinical history.

A history of hypertension or pre-eclampsia during pregnancy makes the subsequent development of essential hypertension much more likely, though it is far from clear why this is so. Similarly, women who have had significant rises in blood pressure when taking the combined oral contraceptive pill are at increased risk of developing hypertension years later, usually when they are post-menopausal.

### Family history

> **The occurrence of hypertension in first-degree relatives greatly increases risk**

As noted previously, the occurrence of hypertension in first-degree relatives greatly increases risk. Evidence may be indirect, especially as blood pressure was little thought about, still less measured, in the generation whose children are now middle aged. This is even more applicable to patients whose families came from other countries, often those with increased hypertension risk such as Jamaica, or from rural areas in the UK or other European countries. A history of stroke, especially in young or middle-aged people, is of course a strong pointer even if nothing is known about blood pressure readings. To a lesser extent this is true of heart and other vascular diseases, though blood sugar and lipid measurements are at least as relevant.

### Social history

> **Patients should be asked to bring their packets of medication every time they are seen in a clinic or surgery**

Several aspects of this have already been discussed: socio-economic class, alcohol, smoking, salt and calorie intake, and drugs, prescribed or otherwise. Of these one can make reasonably confident assessments about only the first of these. This does not mean that one should avoid attempts to define and quantitate the others, just that the results may not be too reliable. With respect to prescribed drugs, including those given for hypertension itself, everyone is familiar with the discrepancies between what we think patients are taking and what they are actually taking (if anything!). Patients should be asked to bring their packets of medication every time they are seen in a clinic or surgery, or at the least the prescription that they are currently taking to be dispensed.

### Physical examination

Although hypertension may produce a variety of clinical signs reflecting the presence of raised blood pressure, it is certainly rare to find physical indicators of a specific underlying cause. Examples where one might be able to take some sort of diagnostic shortcut include:

- cushingoid appearance
- *café au lait* spots suggesting neurofibromatosis and in turn phaeochromocytoma or renovascular disease
- clinically evident hyperthyroidism, which may give rise to raised systolic pressure.

More routinely, the following are crucial parts of the physical assessment.

### Cardiovascular system

- **Blood pressure measurement:** discussed in detail below.
- **Pulse:** rarely a strong pointer either quantitatively or qualitatively but perhaps during paroxysmal rises in phaeochromocytoma when bradycardia may be a helpful clue. On the other hand, a rapid pulse with apparently high pressure is suggestive of a white-coat effect, possibly of hyperthyroidism, or perhaps of sleep apnoea. This too is discussed below.
- **Radiofemoral delay:** this suggests aortic coarctation, which may not be diagnosed till adult life in less severe cases.
- **Cardiac apex:** although the cardiac apex beat may be displaced or unusually forceful in established hypertension, false negatives are very likely and these are certainly not sensitive signs.
- **Heart sounds:** a loud aortic second sound is common in hypertension but is not invariable and has no specific diagnostic or prognostic importance. The same is true of the systolic flow murmurs that also occur and may be quite loud. In the elderly, similar signs may indicate aortic stenosis in the absence of hypertension. Coarctation is likely to produce a widespread and loud systolic murmur, sometimes radiating posteriorly around the edges of the scapula.
- **Bruits:** bruits over the renal arteries (about 5cm above and 10cm lateral to the umbilicus) may be found in the presence of renal artery stenosis but both false positives and negatives are common.
- **Fundi:** the retina provides a direct view of the state of the arterioles in the circulation. It is still common to use the Keith-Wagener classification in describing the appearance of the fundi (Figure 28).

  In fact the vast majority of patents (fortunately) will be in grades 0 (normal), I and II when first diagnosed, so one is working within a rather narrow range of descriptors. However, unequivocal vascular changes are confirmatory evidence for the presence of hypertension when that is in doubt. There is research in progress on more objective quantitative approaches to assessing the fundal vasculature.

*A rapid pulse with apparently high pressure is suggestive of a white-coat effect*

*The retina provides a direct view of the state of the arterioles in the circulation*

### Other systems

Basal rales in the lungs are likely to mean some degree of heart failure, where hypertension may be a significant factor. Enlarged palpable kidneys may be a sign of polycystic disease. There may be signs of hepatic dysfunction in alcohol abuse, though this is more likely associated with hypotension when liver disease is advanced.

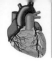

Fig. 28 Keith-Wagener classification describing the appearance of the fundi.

| Grade | Features |
|-------|----------|
| I | Minor narrowing of arterioles |
| II | Increased narrowing and arteriovenous nipping, i.e. compression of venules |
| III | Retinal haemorrhages and/or cotton wool spots (retinal infarcts) and/or hard exudates (leakage of extravascular protein) |
| IV | As in III with papilloedema, the characteristic feature of malignant hypertension |

### Blood pressure measurement

The apparent simplicity of this process has undoubtedly led to the risk, as well as the reality, of complacency. Given the crucial importance of the figures obtained a standardized reproducible technique is essential (Figure 29). The following points are therefore critically important:

*" Aneroid sphygmomanometers are unreliable and should NOT be used "*

- It is essential to use a validated device. The threat of abolition remains for the mercury sphygmomanometer, on rather flimsy health and safety grounds, but at the time of writing it is still available and many physicians and nurses prefer it to electronic devices. If an electronic device is used then it should be one validated by the British Hypertension Society, or a comparable national or international organization (see Appendix 3). Aneroid sphygmomanometers are unreliable and should NOT be used.
- The cuff should have a bladder that encompasses at least 80% of the circumference of the arm (about 12.5–15 x 33cm, for the average adult). Many patients will therefore require a larger size and a few adults a smaller one.
- The forearm should be resting on a flat surface, slightly flexed and externally rotated, at heart level.
- If a manual sphygmomanometer is used the pressure should be inflated to about 30mmHg above that needed to occlude the brachial artery, or the radial artery if palpation is used for preliminary estimation of systolic pressure. The diaphragm of the stethoscope, with light pressure, should be used for auscultation.
- The cuff should be deflated at about 2–3mmHg per second until there is disappearance of the heart sounds (usually described as Korotkoff's phase 5). However, in some patients this may not happen: for instance in pregnant women with increased cardiac

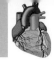

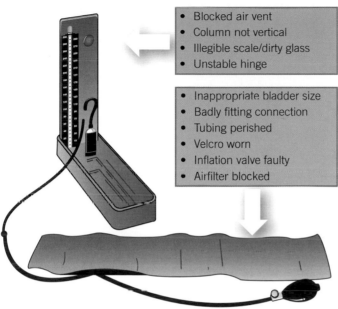

- Blocked air vent
- Column not vertical
- Illegible scale/dirty glass
- Unstable hinge

- Inappropriate bladder size
- Badly fitting connection
- Tubing perished
- Velcro worn
- Inflation valve faulty
- Airfilter blocked

**Fig. 29 Possible sources of error in a sphygmomanometer.**

Reproduced with permission from Slide Atlas of Cardiovascular Risk Factors. Elsevier.

*« Both systolic and diastolic pressures should measured to the nearest 2mmHg NOT to 5mmHg »*

output. In this case phase 4 should be used, when the sounds become muffled, but occasionally even this is difficult to ascertain. If this is used the fact should be noted.

- Both systolic and diastolic pressures should be measured to the nearest 2mmHg NOT to 5mmHg. It is important to avoid parallax error with manual sphygmomanometers, since this can easily amount to 2mmHg.
- At the first consultation the pressure should be measured in both arms in rapid succession. Significant inequalities (> 5mmHg) may indicate aortic coarctation or atherosclerotic narrowing of the axillary artery.
- Note that accurate measurement of blood pressure can be very difficult in the presence of atrial fibrillation, and may require the use of a manual sphygmomanometer rather than an electronic one.
- Blood pressure should be measured at least twice and preferably three times at each visit, with the second and third after the patient has rested for 4–5 minutes. The mean of the last two can be used as the definitive reading but further readings may be needed if the gap between successive observations is greater than 10/6mmHg.
- Unless there is clear evidence of target organ damage at the initial assessment the diagnosis of hypertension should normally be based on three visits several weeks apart.

*« Blood pressure should be measured at least twice and preferably three times at each visit »*

- On the final measurement at the first visit and some or all of the subsequent ones (depending on clinical circumstances) the standing blood pressure should also be measured.

## Investigations
### Routine for all

> *A consistent battery of investigations should form part of the assessment of all new hypertensive patients*

A consistent battery of investigations should form part of the assessment of all new hypertensive patients. These are:

- **Urinalysis:** for protein, blood and glucose, indicating hypertensive renal damage or primary renal disease, as well as possible diabetes.

    There has been much discussion recently concerning micro-albuminuria,[40] that is albumin excretion between 30 and 300mg/24 hours, below the level usually detected by routine dipsticks. Although this finding appears to be associated with increased cardiovascular risk the practical implications are not clear. There is no reason to propose that microalbuminuria should replace conventional risk factors, such as blood pressure itself and lipids, in patient assessment. The targets for intervention continue to be defined in terms of those parameters, not in mg albumin per 24 hours, since that measurement is essentially a marker for vascular damage. At the moment therefore one cannot recommend this assay as a routine procedure: it might encourage more aggressive treatment of other problems but this should happen anyway.

- **Plasma electrolytes and creatinine:** the latter an estimate of renal function, while hypokalaemia may indicate Conn's syndrome or less likely Cushing's syndrome. Sodium levels may be raised under these circumstances. Note that "high" creatinine levels may be entirely normal for patients with large muscle bulk. If there is difficulty in interpreting the figures formal creatinine clearance measurement is indicated.

> *One can expect half of middle-aged hypertensive patients to have Type 2 diabetes*

- **Fasting blood glucose:** one can expect half of middle-aged hypertensive patients to have Type 2 diabetes. Even if not overtly diabetic, patients may have glucose intolerance, and a random blood sugar may detect this or at least indicate the need for further investigation.

- **Fasting lipids:** (if available) should include not only total cholesterol and triglycerides but also LDL and HDL assays to allow a more complete risk assessment. All of these parameters, except triglycerides, can also be usefully measured on random samples but fasting levels are always preferable.

- **Serum uric acid:** up to half of male hypertensive patients may have raised uric acid levels and of course this figure rises in parallel with the creatinine. Clearly these patients are at increased risk of gout if they are subsequently given thiazides. There is controversy about

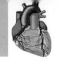

the status of uric acid as a potential cardiovascular risk factor. This issue remains unresolved but an alternative perspective may be that raised uric acid levels represent a defence mechanism, since the compound is a potent endogenous antioxidant. On the other hand, recent evidence has implicated uric acid as a marker for primary as opposed to secondary hypertension in children.

- **Liver function tests:** including gamma-glutamyl transferase (mainly as an index of alcohol intake and abuse).
- **Plasma aldosterone/renin ratio:** almost certainly this will only be available through specialist clinics. It can give a strong pointer towards possible Conn's syndrome and may also give guidance on the initial choice of medication in other cases, as discussed later.
- **Full blood count and ESR:** rarely polycythaemia can be associated with hypertension, while a raised ESR may indicate vasculitis.
- **Electrocardiogram:** the 12-lead ECG may indicate a variety of pathologies but of course is particularly relevant in assessing left ventricular hypertrophy (Figure 20). However, it must be remembered that the sensitivity of the 12-lead ECG is much less than that of echocardiography.

Note that a chest X-ray is not recommended as a routine investigation. It may be useful if coarctation of the aorta is suspected, since there may be notching of some ribs. Naturally there may be other specific indications for chest X-ray, such as possible heart failure. However, it is a very insensitive way of assessing cardiac size.

> *It must be remembered that the sensitivity of the 12-lead ECG is much less than that of echocardiography*

### Selective investigations

A minority of hypertensive patients will require further investigation, though the threshold for extensive investigations is higher than it used to be given the disappointing yield. There are some extremely rare causes of hypertension, usually due to single gene abnormalities, that are so seldom seen, even in tertiary referral centres, that they will not be discussed here. However, some tests will be done relatively frequently, though again usually in specialist centres (see Figure 30 for some indications). Some are for diagnostic purposes, others may be needed later to assess progress.

- **Echocardiography:** not essential in all cases, however, it is valuable in assessing left ventricular mass and structure in patients with borderline hypertension or where the white-coat effect is suspected. It may also be used as a baseline for assessing target organ damage and its possible improvement by antihypertensive treatment. As already noted, it is a much more sensitive measure of left ventricular hypertrophy than the standard ECG. It also serves to assess both diastolic and systolic ventricular function and of

> *A minority of hypertensive patients will require further investigation*

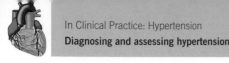
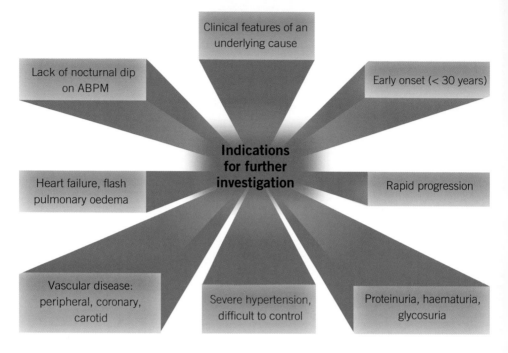

Fig. 30 **Indications for further investigation in hypertension.**

course may detect valve lesions. Unfortunately, the availability of this relatively simple investigation is still shockingly slow in many parts of the UK. Many cardiologists consider magnetic resonance imaging to be preferable, but the problem of availability is even greater, as is the cost.

- *Ambulatory blood pressure monitoring (ABPM):*[41] may also be useful where the diagnosis of hypertension is in doubt. It also gives very useful information on the differential blood pressure profiles during the day and night, which may be particularly helpful in the planning of antihypertensive drug treatments and sometimes gives clues about possible aetiology, such as sleep apnoea.

  The main indications for ABPM are:
  – To assess the extent of a "white-coat" effect.
  – Where blood pressure is very labile or at borderline levels.
  – To assess patients with apparently resistant hypertension.
  – To assess the adequacy of 24-hour blood pressure control, especially when end organ damage appears to progress despite satisfactory clinic readings. This may be particularly important in "non-dippers" whose blood pressure falls little or not all at night (Figure 31).
  – When hypotension is suspected.

*❝ The normal level for ABPM and home readings is lower than for clinic ones ❞*

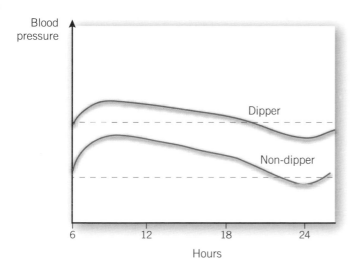

Fig. 31 **Schematic representation of nocturnal "dipping" and "non-dipping" hypertension.**

|  | Systolic (mmHg) | Diastolic (mmHg) |
|---|---|---|
| Surgery/clinic | 140 | 90 |
| 24-hour ambulatory (mean) | 125 | 80 |
| Home (self) | 135 | 85 |

Fig. 32 **Typical variation of blood pressure according to type and place of measurement.**

It should be noted that the normal level for ABPM and home readings is lower than for clinic ones (Figure 32).

However, some individuals have a cuff inflation effect, which raises the blood pressure, and it is obviously impossible to completely escape that except by intra-arterial pressure telemetry, hardly even a semi-routine procedure.

- *Home blood pressure measurements:* provided they are done with well-tested and calibrated machines under clearly specified conditions, are a useful alternative to ABPM for the same indications with the same criteria (although there have been suggestions that thresholds should be about 5mmHg lower) and are also helpful in monitoring the efficacy of treatment since it is obviously impractical (and undesirable) to keep repeating ABPM studies. Clearly there is a fine balance between promoting patient involvement and encouraging excessive, if not obsessive, anxiety: most people involved in hypertension clinics will be familiar with

*❝There is a fine balance between promoting patient involvement and encouraging excessive, if not obsessive, anxiety❞*

47

patients who appear with several pages of figures with perhaps 5 or 6 measurements each day!

66 *Urinary catecholamine measurements are the crucial investigation in the diagnosis of phaeochromocytoma* 99

- *Urinary catecholamine measurements:* are the crucial investigation in the diagnosis of phaeochromocytoma. Traditionally vanillyl mandelic acid (VMA), a catecholamine metabolite, was assayed. Most laboratories now directly measure adrenaline or noradrenaline, or urinary metanephrines, which are thought to be even more sensitive. Slight increases in these compounds may occur with anxiety, thyrotoxicosis or indeed some antihypertensive drugs but in phaeochromocytoma levels are usually several times the upper limit of normal and the diagnosis is seldom in serious doubt. In a few centres, plasma catecholamine measurements are available, and some specialists regard this as more sensitive than any urinary assay. However, it is not universally agreed that this is the case and anyway the issue of availability will almost certainly determine the clinician's choice.

- *Adrenal imaging:* using ultrasound, CT or MRI, will help in the diagnosis of Conn's syndrome, whether due to adenoma or bilateral hyperplasia, and also of phaeochromocytoma. Imaging may be supplemented by selective adrenal vein sampling. The three modalities are listed above in ascending order of sensitivity, cost and waiting time. Although most phaeochromocytomas arise in the adrenal medulla they can be found anywhere where there are sympathetic (chromaffin) neurones, as already noted. Very occasionally these may be localized using a MIBG scan, where a radiolabelled marker that is selectively taken up by chromaffin cells is used.

- *Renovascular investigations:* present some major clinical dilemmas. The "gold standard" remains direct arteriography, a safe but relatively invasive procedure. Magnetic resonance angiography is of course non-invasive, though contrast may be injected intravenously, but produces significant numbers of false negative results. It also needs to be borne in mind that some kidneys with stenotic arteries do not produce excessive amounts of renin and may not actually be contributing to hypertension at all. It is not surprising therefore that this is a controversial area, where experts have very widely differing views. A pragmatic approach would involve consideration of the following:
    - Imaging is essential, or at least highly desirable, in patients with renal bruits, atherosclerosis affecting the legs and with difficult to control hypertension, aged under 30 especially in women, and unexplained raised creatinine.
    - Renal ultrasound may show asymmetrical kidneys, suggesting relative ischaemia on one side, but kidneys with bilateral disease may appear symmetrical and normal in size.

– Reconstruction (stenting or surgery) may normalize blood pressure, especially in young patients with fibromuscular hyperplasia rather than atherosclerosis. If, as is usual, it does not do so, it may still make the blood pressure easier to control, slow down deterioration in renal function, or alternatively may have no effect at all. Ultimately most patients will still need drug therapy.

## Treating hypertension

It is worth emphasizing again, both to ourselves and our patients, that **hypertension is worth treating** (Figure 33). We are preventing or

| Event | Risk reduction |
|---|---|
| Stroke | 28–38 % |
| Coronary heart disease | 16–20 % |
| Congestive heart failure | 16–18 % |

**Fig. 33 Reductions of risk shown in trials of antihypertensive drugs.** Based on trials up to 2003.

minimizing the consequences already discussed. **For successful management of hypertension this needs to be discussed fully with patients, since they are starting a long-term and possibly life-long programme of treatment.** The effect on stroke is of course particularly marked, but, on the whole, the reduction in cardiac events has been less than might have been expected on epidemiological grounds, for reasons that are controversial. Is it because the influence of other risk factors, such as lipids, is not sufficiently taken into account? Or do some of the antihypertensive drugs actually worsen atherosclerosis and accelerate coronary artery disease? In the following discussion it is assumed that in all patients with blood pressure equal to or greater than 140/90mmHg therapeutic intervention is needed, with or without antihypertensive drugs. Although the most accurate approach is to use risk tables or algorithms to determine each individual's level of risk it might be useful to consider the following (Figure 34):

- If the blood pressure is > 180mmHg systolic or > 110mmHg diastolic (grade 3) then drug treatment should be initiated immediately.
- If pressure is grade 1 or 2 and there are no added risk factors and no evidence of target organ damage, suggest lifestyle measures and follow for 3–6 months: if the blood pressure is not <140/90mmHg start drug therapy.

***The reduction in cardiac events has been less than might have been expected on epidemiological grounds**

***The most accurate approach is to use risk tables or algorithms to determine each individual's level of risk**

49

| Target organ damage | Risk factors** | Associated conditions |
|---|---|---|
| • Left ventricular hypertrophy (as assessed by ECG or echocardiogram)<br>• Albuminuria (including microalbuminuria)<br>• Raised serum creatinine<br>• Retinopathy (unequivocal changes)<br>• (Ultrasound evidence of atherosclerosis in carotid or femoral arteries)* | • Age (> 55 years for men, > 65 years for women)<br>• Smoking<br>• Dyslipidaemia<br>• Family history of premature cardiovascular disease<br>• Abdominal obesity (waist circumference: > 102 cm in men, > 88 cm in women)<br>• (C-reactive protein, by high-sensitivity assay)*<br>• (Plasma homocysteine level)* | • Diabetes<br>• Vascular disease at any site<br>• Renal disease regardless of aetiology |

*May be useful but are not routinely available
**Only includes those likely to influence decision on treatment

**Fig. 34 Considerations in deciding to start antihypertensive therapy.**

- If there is **any** indication of target organ damage start drug therapy without delay.
- If **any** risk factors or associated conditions are present consider drug treatment without delay – **always in diabetic patients** – but this should always be the case if there are more than two such factors or conditions.
- If blood pressure is in the high normal range drug treatment should be started in patients with diabetes and/or impaired renal function.

### Non-pharmacological approaches[5,6]

Hypertension is a chronic, indeed usually a life-long disorder. It is therefore understandable that many people will seek alternatives to years or even decades of drug treatment and the health professionals advising them should not be dismissive of this wish nor of the importance of lifestyle and other non-pharmacological measures. The list of potential non-pharmacological therapies is a long one and some are listed in Figure 35. However, although several of these interventions are desirable and well-founded in terms of clinical evidence, it is only realistic to recognize that many patients will not adhere to them and that in any case their efficacy is usually limited. A

*" Many people will seek alternatives to years or even decades of drug treatment "*

---

### Non-pharmacological interventions

*Measures that lower blood pressure*
- weight reduction
- decrease salt intake
- decrease alcohol consumption
- increase physical exercise

*Measures to reduce cardiovascular risk*
- stop smoking
- decrease intake of saturated fat and increase poly- and mono-unsaturates
- increase oily fish consumption
- reduce total fat intake
- increase fruit and vegetable consumption (related to increased potassium intake?)

---

particularly important example is weight reduction, given that some though not all patients have blood pressures that are extremely sensitive to changes in body weight. Salt reduction is also difficult to achieve with sufficient rigour, if indeed this is a worthwhile objective (see previous discussion).

In fact, most patients will require drug therapy. The non-drug approach most likely to yield results is weight loss and this should always be encouraged and supported by detailed dietary advice. Of course, the potential benefits are not restricted to blood pressure reduction. In fact, the association of overweight with the development of diabetes is probably a more important global risk factor: global for the individual patient but also from the point of view of public health. It is vital that non-pharmacological strategies are not abandoned when drug treatment is initiated, though many patients and some clinicians may feel that it is safe and convenient to do so.

Particular comment is appropriate with regard to weight reducing drugs: although a matter of pharmacology they are also part of the overall approach to weight reduction. At the time of writing two drugs are licensed as adjuvant therapies for weight reduction: orlistat and sibutramine.[42] These work in totally different ways. Orlistat blocks the digestion of fats (triglycerides) in the lumen of the gut and is hardly absorbed into the systemic circulation. Sibutramine, on the other hand, acts centrally to suppress appetite and has a pharmacological profile similar to some antidepressants, such as venlafaxine, in inhibiting uptake of noradrenaline and serotonin at central synapses. There is clinical trial evidence for the efficacy of both drugs and this is not the

**Fig. 35 Non-pharmacological measures in hypertensive patients.**

*66The non-drug approach most likely to yield results is weight loss 99*

place for detailed comparisons. However it should be noted that sibutramine can cause modest increases in heart rate and blood pressure (2–3mmHg), though the latter is generally cancelled out if there is successful weight loss.

*** Sibutramine can cause modest increases in heart rate and blood pressure ***

## Available drug therapies: pros and cons

Compared with 20, or even 10, years ago, today's prescriber has a huge choice of antihypertensive agents (Figure 36). This does not make

Fig. 36 Classes of antihypertensive drugs

| Class | Examples |
|---|---|
| **Diuretics** • Thiazides • Loop diuretics | Bendroflumethiazide (bendrofluazide) Furosemide (frusemide) |
| **Beta-blockers** • Non-vasodilator • Vasodilator | Atenolol, bisoprolol Labetalol, pindolol, nebivolol |
| **Calcium-channel blockers** • dihydropyridines • heart rate limiting | Amlodipine Diltiazem, verapamil |
| **ACE inhibitors** | Lisinopril, perindopril |
| **Angiotensin II receptor antagonists** | Losartan, candesartan |
| **Alpha-blockers** | Doxazosin |
| **Aldosterone-receptor blockers** | Spironolactone |
| **Centrally acting drugs** | Moxonidine |
| **Miscellaneous vasodilators** | Hydrallazine, minoxidil |

decisions any easier, particularly since views on specific drug classes can change remarkably quickly. Figure 37 briefly summarizes the discussion in this section. There are other drugs used only in emergencies or urgencies, such as sodium nitroprusside and intravenous glyceryl trinitrate, and these will be discussed later. In

| Class of drug | Conditions favouring use | Contraindications | Side effects |
|---|---|---|---|
| Diuretics (usually thiazides, maybe loop) | Heart failure, age > 60 years, isolated systolic hypertension, African origin | Gout, pregnancy (relative) | Hypokalaemia, hyperuricaemia, glucose intolerance, hypercalcaemia (thiazides), dyslipidaemia, hyponatraemia, impotence (thiazides) |
| Beta-blockers (without vasodilator properties) * | Angina, previous MI, tachyarrhythmias, migraine, anxiety | Asthma, chronic obstructive pulmonary disease, 2nd/3rd degree heart block Peripheral vascular disease (relative) | Bronchospasm, bradycardia, heart failure, cold extremities, insomnia or vivid dreams, fatigue, decreased exercise tolerance, dyslipidaemia, impaired glucose tolerance, impotence |
| ACE inhibitors | Heart failure, left ventricular dysfunction, previous MI, diabetic or other nephropathy, proteinuria | Pregnancy, bilateral renal-artery stenosis, hyperkalaemia | Cough, angioedema (rare), hyperkalaemia, rash, distortion of taste |
| Calcium-channel blockers | Age > 60, systolic hypertension, ciclosporin-induced hypertension, peripheral vascular disease | Heart block (verapamil, diltiazem) Uncontrolled heart failure | Headache, flushing, gingival hyperplasia, ankle oedema, paradoxical angina |
| Alpha-blockers | Prostatic hyperplasia, dyslipidaemia | Orthostatic hypotension, fatigue | Headache, drowsiness, fatigue, weakness, postural hypotension |
| Angiotensin II receptor antagonists | ACE inhibitor associated cough or angioedema, diabetic or other nephropathy, proteinuria, congestive heart failure | Pregnancy, bilateral renal-artery stenosis, hyperkalaemia | Angioedema (very rare), cough (rare) |
| Aldosterone-receptor blockers | Heart failure, previous MI, resistant hypertension | Renal insufficiency, hyperkalaemia | Hyperkalaemia, gynaecomastia, menstrual irregularity |

**Fig. 37**
**Antihypertensive drugs: potential indications, contraindications and adverse effects.** * Beta-blockers with vasodilator properties: carvedilol, labetalol, nebivolol.

*" Today's prescriber has a huge choice of antihypertensive agents "*

addition there are a number of vasodilators used only in very resistant hypertension in exceptional circumstances and therefore these will not be discussed further here. Minoxidil is the best known of these (though perhaps better known as a hair restorer for bald men!). Diazoxide is used even less frequently: its main use is treating inoperable insulinomas where it inhibits insulin release.

## Diuretics (especially thiazides)
### Mechanism of action

*Thiazide diuretics are among the longest established and probably the most extensively tested antihypertensive drugs*

Although thiazide diuretics are among the longest established and probably the most extensively tested antihypertensive drugs, we still have a very poor understanding of their mechanism of action. As might be expected, they produce both volume depletion and sodium loss at first, accompanied by a fall in peripheral resistance (sometimes briefly preceded by an increase) and cardiac output. With chronic use (more than a couple of months) lowered peripheral resistance and increased sodium excretion persist, but cardiac output and blood volume gradually return to pre-treatment amounts. A direct vasodilator effect is almost certainly relevant at this stage and later, but has proved difficult to demonstrate unequivocally except *in vitro* using high concentrations of the drugs. Loop diuretics may also be useful, especially in people with significant fluid overload.

Spironolactone and eplerenone, respectively old and new antagonists of the aldosterone receptor (the latter not yet available in the UK), have found an increased role in the management of resistant hypertension, as will be discussed later.

### Advantages
- Very good evidence of efficacy and long-term reduction in stroke and cardiovascular events, especially in the elderly. This has been reinforced recently, and somewhat controversially, by the publication of the US ALLHAT study and by a meta-analysis of over 40 clinical trials.
- Negligible cost.
- Convenient dosage regimen.

### Disadvantages
- Potential metabolic abnormalities – hypokalaemia and hypo-natraemia, hyperuricaemia, impaired glucose tolerance, worsening lipid profile, hypomagnesaemia (apart perhaps from hyper-uricaemia, these can be minimized by low doses and hypokalaemia specifically by concurrent potassium-sparing diuretics, such as amiloride or spironolactone, or by ACE inhibitors).
- May cause worsening of glucose tolerance and of lipid profile, with reduction in HDL cholesterol and increase in triglycerides (this is largely absent with indapamide).
- May cause postural hypotension.
- May cause impotence – a problem with any blood pressure lowering drug but almost certainly worse with thiazides for unknown reasons.
- Very rare liver, bone marrow and skin toxicity.

## Beta-blockers
### Mechanism of action
Once again, the exact mechanism of action of these very well-established drugs is uncertain, but the general view is that lowering of blood pressure is associated with diminished cardiac output in the presence of peripheral resistance that may actually increase: pure beta-blockers are not vasodilators. For drugs with partial agonist activity (so-called intrinsic sympathomimetic activity, or ISA), such as pindolol, there may, however, be some fall in peripheral resistance with a less marked reduction in cardiac output, probably caused by vasodilatation. Some other beta-blockers have definite vasodilator activity from alpha$_1$-adrenergic blockade (labetalol) or have a direct action on smooth muscle by enhancing nitric oxide release (nebivolol). In this case vasodilatation may be a contributory element in the fall in blood pressure but the overall reduction in blood pressure is not greater than with the conventional beta-blockers. We do not have direct comparison with regards to clinical outcomes, the large trials having almost universally involved non-vasodilating beta-blockers. It must also be remembered that beta-blockers also cause a lowering in renin secretion, which can contribute significantly to blood pressure reduction in patients with high-renin hypertension: as noted, such patients are usually relatively young. Contrary to statements in some textbooks, hypotension can be dangerously abrupt if such patients are given a beta-blocker, especially if they have previously been exposed to a potent vasodilator such as a calcium-channel blocker.

> **"Pure beta-blockers are not vasodilators"**

> **"Beta-blockers also cause a lowering in renin secretion"**

### Advantages
- Long-term efficacy and beneficial effects on morbidity and mortality are well proven in trials.
- Useful in patients with co-existing angina.
- Useful in some anxious patients.
- Usually simple once-daily dosing.

### Disadvantages
- Can cause sinus bradycardia and precipitate heart block.
- Can precipitate or aggravate heart failure because of an inhibitory effect on cardiac contractility (negative inotropy), though also a key part of the mechanism of action, in heart failure as well as hypertension.
- Can cause dangerous bronchospasm in patients with asthma or chronic obstructive pulmonary disease.

- May cause deterioration in peripheral vascular disease – of doubtful relevance in atherosclerosis with intermittent claudication, but important in Raynaud's phenomenon.
- Can worsen lipid profile and impair insulin sensitivity (less marked or absent with drugs with ISA, alpha-blocking or other vasodilator properties).
- May decrease awareness of hypoglycaemia in diabetics (again of dubious clinical importance, though much quoted!).
- Can cause sleep disturbance, including nightmares.
- May precipitate or aggravate depression.

### Calcium-channel blockers
#### Mechanism of action

*66 Calcium-channel blockers are a large and fairly heterogeneous group of drugs with differing properties 99*

This is a large and fairly heterogeneous group of drugs with differing properties. As far as their hypotensive effect is concerned, however, it is likely to be the vasodilator effect that is crucial, with inhibition of calcium entry into blood vessels leading to reduced smooth muscle tone in arterioles and therefore reduced peripheral resistance.

#### Advantages
- Short-term efficacy good, some outcome data available especially in the elderly.
- May be useful in angina (especially non-dihydropyridines, or dihydropyridines if combined with beta-blockers).
- Few absolute contraindications (e.g. safe in asthma, peripheral vascular disease).
- Simple dosage regimens, though sometimes only with modified-release preparations.
- Proven efficacy in isolated systolic hypertension (long-acting dihydropyridine).

#### Disadvantages
- May cause flushing, headache, ankle oedema (especially dihydropyridines, though there may be within-class differences even among those).
- May cause reflex sympathetic activation secondary to vasodilatation (especially short-acting dihydropyridines, which should not be used at all): tachycardia, possible long-term adverse effects on cardiac events and mortality.
- May cause bradycardia and negative inotropy, in case of non-dihydropyridines, therefore caution in impaired left ventricular function.
- Rare gum hyperplasia (particularly dihydropyridines). Note that phenytoin also has calcium-channel blocking properties.

## Angiotensin converting enzyme (ACE) inhibitors and angiotensin II receptor antagonists (AIIRAs)
### Mechanisms of action

Angiotensin II can raise blood pressure by several mechanisms, including the potentiation of sympathetic action (Figure 38). It is not surprising, therefore, that inhibition of angiotensin II formation, or antagonism of vascular angiotensin II receptors (specifically the AT1 subtype), will lower blood pressure when there is high renin activity. It is perhaps more interesting and unexpected that these drugs are also effective in some patients with normal or low renin levels. One plausible reason is the fact that ACE inhibitors also affect other enzymes, notably kininase, which is involved in the breakdown of vasodilator peptides such as bradykinin and substance P (and is in fact the same molecule as angiotensin converting enzyme). In theory this should not apply to the AIIRAs though recent data suggest that increased bradykinin release may occur

> *ACE inhibitors also affect other enzymes, notably kininase, which is involved in the breakdown of vasodilator peptides such as bradykinin and substance P*

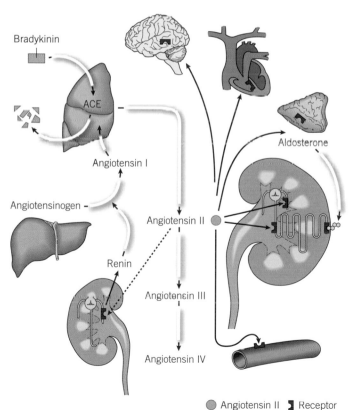

Bradykinin

ACE

Angiotensin I

Angiotensinogen

Aldosterone

Angiotensin II

Renin

Angiotensin III

Angiotensin IV

● Angiotensin II ❱ Receptor

**Fig. 38 Formation of angiotensins and organs affected by their actions.** Reproduced with permission from Goodfriend et al. angiotensin receptors and their antagonists. N Engl J Med 1996;334:1649–54. Copyright © 1996 Massachusetts Medical Society. All rights reserved.

because of the effect of increased levels of angiotensin II on the other angiotensin receptor, AT2, which in turn is linked to kinin synthesis.

### Advantages
- Effective in most patient groups (but see below).
- May provide specific renal protection in diabetes with or without hypertension.
- Safe in most patients (but see below).
- Long duration of action especially for newer agents (e.g. trandolapril and perindopril).
- Enhanced well-being reported in some studies – possible cognitive improvement or at least slowing of cognitive deterioration?
- AIIRAs exceptionally well-tolerated, even better than ACE inhibitors and best of all currently available agents.

### Disadvantages
- First-dose hypotension, especially in sodium and volume-depleted patients: uncommon with longer-acting agents (e.g. perindopril and trandolapril) and the AIIRAs, and probably overemphasized in everyday clinical practice. It is more likely to occur in patients with heart failure on high doses of diuretics.
- Irritating dry cough in 5–20% of patients, sometimes causing discontinuation of the drug: much less common with the AIIRAs but can still occur.
- May rarely cause anaphylactoid reactions (angioedema) (<1%): also very uncommonly occurs with the AIIRAs.
- Deterioration in renal function in patients with renovascular disease, due to altered intrarenal haemodynamics – this can be severe and may lead rapidly to renal failure in the presence of bilateral disease. It is possible that the AIIRAs can cause similar problems but this has yet to be fully assessed.
- ACE inhibitors alone have limited efficacy in black hypertensives with low or suppressed renin levels. The same is true of most elderly patients from any ethnic group. Response to the AIIRAs may be better but the issue is controversial.
- The occurrence of breakthrough with ACE inhibitors, a secondary loss of response to these drugs after months or years of efficacy, possibly associated with increased synthesis of angiotensin II by pathways not inhibited by ACE inhibitors.
- Both drug types are absolutely contraindicated in pregnancy due to teratogenicity.

*" ACE inhibitors and AIIRAs are absolutely contraindicated in pregnancy "*

## Alpha$_1$-blockers
### Mechanism of action

The principal mode of action of these drugs is inhibition of noradrenaline-induced vasoconstriction by blocking alpha$_1$-adrenergic receptors in the vascular wall. There may also be some central inhibition of sympathetic activity, though this may be more important in preventing reflex tachycardia than in lowering blood pressure.

*"The principal mode of action of alpha$_1$-blockers is inhibition of noradrenaline-induced vasoconstriction"*

### Advantages
- Once-daily dosage for newer compounds (e.g. doxazosin).
- Few contraindications.
- Neutral or possibly beneficial metabolic effects, especially on lipid profile: reduced total cholesterol, but more especially increased HDL cholesterol.

### Disadvantages
- May cause postural hypotension, particularly first-dose effect (less likely with new longer-acting agents).
- Can cause tiredness and sedation.
- Dose may need to be titrated over a broad range if used as monotherapy: in fact it is not regarded by most specialists as suitable for that role.

## Centrally acting drugs, or sympatholytics
### Mechanism of action

These drugs reduce sympathetic outflow at the level of the brainstem but not all by the same mechanisms. Reserpine, the oldest of these drugs (and one of the oldest drugs in use for any purpose), depletes neurones of noradrenaline and other monoamine neurotransmitters. Methyldopa and clonidine act primarily as agonists at inhibitory pre-synaptic alpha$_2$-adrenergic receptors. The newer drugs moxonidine and rilmenidine (not available in the UK) are believed to be relatively selective agonists at imidazoline $I_1$ receptors in the rostral ventrolateral medulla, the region regulating sympathetic outflow.

### Advantages
- Long experience of efficacy, including long-term outcome studies (reserpine).
- Simple dosage (except with methyldopa).
- Convenient dosage in modified-release form (in some countries for clonidine), or as conventional formulation (moxonidine).
- Very low cost (at least for reserpine and methyldopa).
- Known to be safe in pregnancy (methyldopa).

*"Methyldopa is known to be safe in pregnancy"*

- No adverse effects in asthma.
- Possible improvement in glucose tolerance (moxonidine)?

### Disadvantages
- Can cause sedation and depression, sometimes severe (reserpine, methyldopa).
- May cause sodium and water retention (less with moxonidine, rilmenidine).
- Dry mouth.
- May cause parkinsonian syndrome (methyldopa).
- Hyperprolactinaemia – galactorrhoea, impotence, menstrual disturbance (methyldopa).
- Sometimes causes liver damage, haemolytic anaemia (methyldopa).
- Rebound hypertension (clonidine especially – much less likely with modified-release formulations, not reported so far with imidazoline agonists).

## Targets and guidelines: how successful are we?

There is increasing international consensus on targets for treatment (Figure 39). Given the greatly expanded range of therapies available, as

Fig. 39 International consensus on blood pressure targets.

| Consensus blood pressure targets | |
| --- | --- |
| General target | < 140/85 mmHg |
| Patients with diabetes, renal impairment or proteinuria | < 130/80 mmHg |
| *Ideally 10 mmHg less, if achievable, in both categories* | |

well as the emphasis on individualized approaches to selecting medication, the above question is a very reasonable one. It is made more acute by the increasingly ambitious targets set by bodies such as the European Society of Hypertension and the US Joint National Committee. The British Hypertension Society has recently published its own guidelines, which are largely in line with the European ones, with some variations that will be mentioned at relevant points in the text.[43]

*" More intensive therapy was associated with better results "*

There are now extensive data from many countries. The results are discouraging, to say the least. A recent US study of 800 hypertensive men with a mean age of about 65 years showed that 40% had blood pressure above 160/90mmHg despite six or more clinic visits a year in excellent centres,[44] and over 75% had blood pressure greater than 140/90mmHg. As might be expected, more intensive therapy, as judged by the frequency of increases in the number of drugs or their dose, was associated with better results. The most recent survey in five European countries, Canada and the USA was not much more encouraging:[45] about 29% of American and 17% of Canadian patients had well controlled blood pressure of at most 140/90mmHg but in European countries (England, Germany, Sweden, Italy and Spain) the figure is 10% or less. It has to be noted though that these data are already several years old despite recent publication. Although the rather clichéd rule of halves may no longer be wholly applicable, improvement seems due mostly to better detection and greater awareness of hypertension: treatment is generally *not* more successful in those who are identified as hypertensive. Why not? Obviously there is no single answer but the following issues are likely to be relevant:

*66Improvement seems due mostly to better detection and greater awareness of hypertension 99*

- Clinicians may be satisfied with modest improvements in blood pressure and fail to pursue targets, even when they claim otherwise: the "something is better than nothing" approach. The Cardiomonitor study[46] is particularly revealing in this respect: although 95% of patients and 76% of doctors thought hypertension was controlled, in fact blood pressure was below 160/90mmHg in only 37% of cases!
- The drug may not be the optimal choice from the outset, and additions or replacements may be similarly inappropriate.
- Secondary hypertension may not be recognized, and contributory problems such as obesity may not be successfully managed, or managed at all. This is also a contributory factor in resistant or refractory hypertension.
- Patients do not continue (or even may not start) treatment: failure to understand the reasons for it, resistance to the idea of long-term drug therapy, they cannot afford the cost of treatment or because of drug side effects.

As an indication of the size of the problem, a large survey of hypertensive patients in general practices in the UK, in 1995,[47] showed that 40 to 50% of patients discontinued their initial medication within 6 months, irrespective of the class of drug involved. However, more recent data on the ACE inhibitors and the AIIRAs have been more positive,[48] suggesting 12-month continuation rates of about 69%, including a figure of 75% for ACE inhibitors and AIIRAs, 71% for calcium-channel blockers, 68% for diuretics, 64% for beta-blockers, and 59% for alpha-blockers and other miscellaneous drugs. In most patients the drug was altered to one from another class, though it was not clear whether efficacy or side effects was the stronger determinant in such a change. About one-third of the cost of treating hypertension can be attributed to patients who switch or discontinue therapy.

*66About one-third of the cost of treating hypertension can be attributed to patients who switch or discontinue therapy 99*

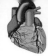

## Monotherapy: choosing the first line of treatment

*Patients and doctors would certainly prefer to use single drug therapy*

If drug treatment of hypertension is considered necessary, patients and doctors would certainly prefer to use single drug therapy. This is increasingly seen as unrealistic. Before discussing the reasons for this in detail it is worth noting two now classic US studies that compared several major classes of antihypertensive agents and to consider the previously mentioned meta-analysis of outcomes of a large number of trials published in the last decade.

The Treatment of Mild Hypertension Study (TOMHS)[49] enrolled over 900 middle-aged men with diastolic blood pressures between 90 and 99mmHg, who were randomly assigned to placebo or one of the following: the beta-blocker acebutolol; the calcium-channel blocker amlodipine; the thiazide diuretic chlorthalidone; the alpha-blocker doxazosin; or the ACE inhibitor enalapril. All the treatments were more effective than placebo in lowering systolic and diastolic blood pressure but the differences between them were small, spanning a 3.3mmHg range for systolic pressure and a 2.5mmHg range for diastolic pressure. After correction for placebo this represented a range from 2.7 to 6.0mmHg reduction for systolic and 1.1 to 3.6mmHg for diastolic pressure. In fact, given the within-group variability these were not significant differences. Effects on other variables, such as left ventricular mass and ECG abnormalities, also failed to reveal important differences.

*The authors concluded that treatment had to be tailored to the individual patient*

The Veterans Administration Co-operative Study Group[50] compared six agents with placebo: hydrochlorothiazide, atenolol, captopril, the centrally acting sympatholytic drug clonidine, prazosin, and a modified-release formulation of diltiazem. The trial recruited nearly 1300 men, just under half of whom were black, who had diastolic blood pressures between 95 and 109mmHg. Once again all treatments were clearly superior to placebo, but in this study there were some apparent differences in efficacy. Overall, diltiazem was the most effective in terms of blood pressure reduction, at least as regards diastolic pressure, and was effective in reducing diastolic pressure below 90mmHg in 75% of treated patients. The other drugs produced response rates, by the above criterion, between 54% and 65%, while placebo produced responses in 33% of patients. Perhaps more importantly, the authors concluded that treatment had to be tailored to the individual patient (while recognizing that their data could not necessarily be extrapolated to women). Incidentally, they noted that captopril and atenolol, which tend to suppress renin levels, were more effective in younger than older white men, while in blacks of all ages diltiazem produced the best response. This finding was consistent with the

*Black and older white hypertensives tend to have low or even suppressed renin levels*

previously reported observations that black and older white hypertensives tend to have low or even suppressed renin levels and tended to respond better to drugs such as thiazides and calcium-channel blockers that actually increase renin levels but lower blood pressure by other mechanisms.[51] There is further support for this in a recent, much smaller study from Cambridge, in which there was clearly superior efficacy for monotherapy with ACE inhibitors and beta-blockers in younger men.

A recent meta-analysis concluded that low-dose diuretics were at least equal to any other form of drug therapy in terms of blood pressure reduction and, more importantly, with respect to clinical outcomes.[52] It is difficult to analyse all components of the study, but the other broad conclusion appears to be that blood pressure lowering medication of all types reduces the risk of cardiovascular events.

The enormous ALLHAT study (the Antihypertensive and Lipid-Lowering treatment to prevent Heart Attack Trial),[53] involved over 40,000 patients randomized to chlorthalidone, amlodipine, lisinopril, atenololol and, initially, to doxazosin – the latter arm was stopped prematurely because of a concern of increased risk of the development of heart failure. The overall conclusion was that chlorthalidone, or presumably by extension other diuretics, should be the first-line therapy in primary hypertension. In fact this has formed the basis of the JNC7 recommendations. The trial's design and interpretation has evoked enormous controversy, and European reaction has been largely unfavourable for several reasons, including the overwhelming primacy given to diuretics as first-line therapy. In contrast an Australian study (ANBP2)[54] of some 6000 patients over the age of 65 years directly compared diuretics and ACE inhibitors as first line therapy, with add-on drugs as needed, and concluded the latter were superior in preventing cardiovascular events with equivalent lowering of blood pressure. This confusing discrepancy has recently been reviewed as part of what has understandably been called the "alphabetic maze of recent studies".[55] In fact it may be more apparent than real, reflecting different patient populations.[56]

In clinical practice, there is general consensus that monotherapy may achieve target blood pressures in 50–60% of patients at most, though published trials for individual drugs are often more optimistic. This view has been reinforced by several important trials, which will be discussed later. It is also very important to remember that most antihypertensive drug side effects are dose related, with the probable exception of ACE inhibitors (cough and angioedema).

Despite this, it is still very relevant to attempt a rational choice of initial drug therapy. The principal bases for this must be (Figure 40):

*There was clearly superior efficacy for monotherapy with ACE inhibitors and beta-blockers in younger men*

*Blood pressure lowering medication of all types reduces the risk of cardiovascular events*

*Monotherapy may achieve target blood pressures in 50–60% of patients at most*

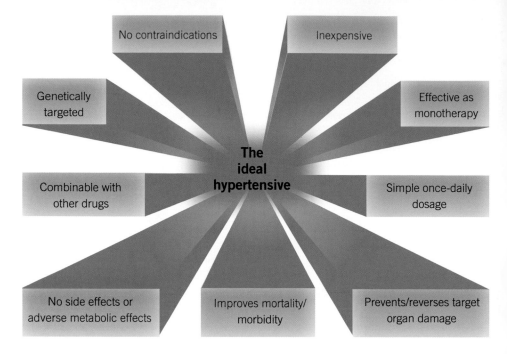

Fig. 40 Properties of the ideal antihypertensive agent.

- On the positive side, there may be trial evidence that the drug is likely to be particularly effective in a given patient. Some of these considerations have been mentioned previously. There is very substantial evidence, for instance, for the efficacy of the thiazides in the elderly, as well as for known ethnic differences in response. There are also concurrent diseases that can affect the choice of medication and provide more or less compelling grounds for choosing particular drugs.
- On the negative side, there may be equally compelling reasons why a drug should be avoided in individual patients. Some issues still remain controversial, notably the role of dihydropyridine calcium-channel blockers in diabetic hypertensives. At present the general view is that long-acting agents of this type are not harmful and may be beneficial, especially in terms of renoprotection and even more so when combined with ACE inhibitors, but unfortunately the quality of much of the data is disappointing. Certainly, the excessive anxiety about these drugs has subsided in the last couple of years.

A practical approach to drug selection has been proposed by Morris Brown and his colleagues in Cambridge.[57] It is based on the so-called ABCD classification and has been adopted as a formal recommendation by the British Hypertension Society, which has been reinforced in their recently published guidelines (Figure 41):

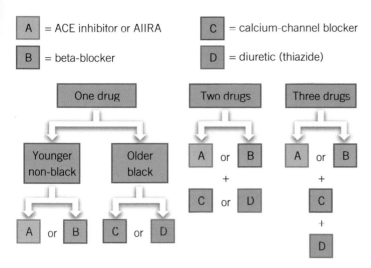

A = ACE inhibitor or AIIRA

B = beta-blocker

C = calcium-channel blocker

D = diuretic (thiazide)

**Fig. 41 The ABCD system for choosing antihypertensive therapy.** Ref. 57.

*66All the major classes of antihypertensive drugs may be considered as first-line therapies 99*

A: ACE inhibitors and AIIRAs

B: beta-blockers

C: calcium-channel blockers

D: diuretics (usually thiazides)

The major distinction between them in terms of mechanism centres on their effects on the renin-angiotensin system:

A and B **reduce** the activity of the system at some point.

C and D **increase** activity but reduce blood pressure by vasodilatation.

Broadly A and B are more appropriate for younger patients (below the age of 50 or 55) while C and D are more effective in the older patients and in black patients of all ages. This naturally has to be considered in the context of the individual's clinical circumstances, as already outlined. The main issue, discussed in the next section, is how soon should we consider the use of combination therapies. However, it is important to appreciate that the consensus in the UK and in Europe generally is that all the major classes of antihypertensive drugs may be considered as first-line therapies, depending on the individual circumstances.

*66Communication between doctor and patients is vital99*

## Combination therapy in hypertension

It is clear that we have nothing like ideal or even acceptable blood pressure control, even though perfect control at a population level is obviously unattainable and we are doing better both in the UK and worldwide than we used to. It is always very easy to say how useless our efforts are, but an over-negative approach is discouraging rather than the opposite. Still, what can be done about it? As always in clinical medicine, communication between doctor and patients is vital, if not always as readily attainable as both would like. We must also try not to miss underlying causes of hypertension, though as already pointed out these may not always lead to cure even if identified, and to take our own targets seriously (we all know how tempting it may be not to do so).

> *About two-thirds of patients needed two or more drugs to attain blood pressures of around 140/85mmHg*

In addition, clinicians might consider the following:

- Try to choose initial therapy rationally, taking into account the points already noted.
- Consider newly introduced drugs, even though the information available may be rather sparse, but most definitely not at the expense of established agents for which evidence is more extensive, and which do work in most patients.
- Consider combination therapy, either free combinations using two or more agents chosen by the clinician, or with fixed-dose formulations. In this context it is now well known that in the Hypertension Optimal Treatment (HOT) study[58] and the United Kingdom Prospective Diabetes Study (UKPDS)[59] about two-thirds of patients needed two or more drugs to attain blood pressures of around 140/85mmHg.

### The rational basis for combination therapy

> *Most antihypertensive drugs can be combined*

What are we hoping to gain from combination therapies in hypertension? The case for combination therapy has both a theoretical and a practical basis. Most antihypertensive drugs can be combined, and there are relatively few cases in which a particular combination is inappropriate or hazardous. They may then:

- complement each other in terms of efficacy, because of differing modes of action producing additive or sometimes even synergistic effects
- counteract each others side effects
- have both of these properties.

In several of the examples quoted below, drugs in combination are balancing counter-regulatory systems that may tend to oppose reductions in blood pressure due to one of the agents acting alone: for instance, thiazides and ACE inhibitors.

Since we do know that essential hypertension is a heterogeneous condition, even if we do not have a very good understanding of the nature of the heterogeneity, in practical terms, therefore, we are looking for:

- increased efficacy, with greater numbers of patients achieving target blood pressures

- no more and preferably fewer side effects and improved quality of life
- improved compliance because of fewer adverse effects
- improved target organ protection
- no significant extra cost, or even reduced cost(!).

The ABCD approach has been applied and the following are considered particularly useful combinations:

A + C

A + D

B + C

but not B + D, particularly in older patients, for reasons already summarized. It should be noted that alpha blockers and centrally acting drugs do not fall within this classification and can usually be added to drugs from other classes as second- or third-line medication.

### Combinations that are actually useful in practice

In fact, most of the ones one would expect. It will not be particularly helpful to consider all possible combinations, but the most widely used ones will be discussed here (see Ref. 60 for full references).

### ACE inhibitors and thiazides, or thiazide-related diuretics

This is one of the best-established combinations, both as free combinations and in fixed-dose formulations. In fact, the latter are the most common fixed-dose combination antihypertensive products worldwide. There is a strong pharmacological case for this combination.

- Both drugs reduce peripheral resistance but by quite different mechanisms (in the case of thiazides, rather obscure ones as has already been noted).
- Thiazides activate the renin-angiotensin system while ACE inhibitors reduce the formation of angiotensin II, its principal product.
- ACE inhibitors will counteract thiazide-induced hypokalaemia by reducing aldosterone secretion and probably also by the reduced direct effect of angiotensin II on renal tubules. They may also reduce hyperuricaemia caused by the thiazides.
- ACE inhibitors enhance the natriuretic action of the thiazides, though this is probably not of major importance in long-term blood pressure reduction.

A particularly important role for this combination is in groups of hypertensive patients with low renin levels, notably Afro-Caribbean and US blacks.

*❝Thiazides activate the renin-angiotensin system while ACE inhibitors reduce the formation of angiotensin II❞*

> *Both drugs may protect renal function in diabetic hypertensives*

Similar considerations apply to the combination of AIIRAs with thiazides and this combination has also become frequently used in the relatively short time that the AIIRAs have been available.

ACE inhibitors and dihydropyridine calcium-channel blockers
These two types of drug are essentially peripheral vasodilators, but act by entirely different mechanisms. There are also other considerations that favour this combination:

- Dihydropyridines tend to activate both the sympathetic nervous system and the renin-angiotensin system, which can potentially blunt their antihypertensive effect: both these effects will be counteracted by ACE inhibition.
- Both drugs promote increased sodium excretion.
- Dihydropyridine-induced ankle oedema, perhaps the single most common reason why patients discontinue these drugs, seems to be diminished by ACE inhibitors.
- Both drugs may protect renal function in diabetic hypertensives, perhaps in an additive manner.

It must be reiterated that short-acting dihydropyridines have no place at all in the acute or chronic management of hypertension, or indeed anything else.

> *Verapamil and diltiazem tend to cause much less sympathetic activation than the dihydropyridines*

ACE inhibitors and non-dihydropyridine calcium-channel blockers
Most of the same points as above are relevant, although calcium-channel blockers such as verapamil and diltiazem tend to cause much less sympathetic activation than the dihydropyridines, and in fact usually reduce heart rate. They also cause less ankle oedema than the dihydropyridines.

> *Short-acting dihydropyridines have no place at all in the acute or chronic management of hypertension*

Beta-blockers and dihydropyridine calcium-channel blockers
This combination is a different situation, since the mode of action of the two drugs is radically different. Beta-blockers do not generally reduce peripheral resistance, and sometimes the contrary occurs. There are several potential advantages:

- Beta-blockers reduce sympathetic activation associated with the calcium-channel blockers.
- Beta-blockers block the increased renin release caused by vasodilatation.
- Calcium-channel blockers counteract the vasoconstriction that may occur with most beta-blockers.

Beta-blockers and thiazides
This combination will be familiar to anyone accustomed to the stepped-care approach of the 1970s, when these were the principal

classes of drugs available. Most clinical outcome data in hypertension, at least until the mid-1990s, have been obtained with one or both of these two classes of drugs. They too complement each other:

- Diuretics increase renin secretion, partly by promoting natriuresis and partly, probably, by vasodilatation.
- Beta-blockers inhibit renin secretion.

However, not all their interactions are favourable. In particular, both drugs may have dose-related adverse effects on the lipid profile, by increasing triglyceride levels and reducing concentrations of HDL cholesterol. It is also possible that they will worsen glucose tolerance and insulin sensitivity, at least with a conventional beta-blocker. In theory this may worsen atherosclerosis, though the clinical relevance is unproven.

### Calcium-channel blockers (dihydropyridines) and alpha-blockers

This is another situation in which two different types of vasodilator are used together. Potentially, there could be increased postural hypotension but in practice this is rarely a problem. Neither class of drug produces adverse metabolic effects.

### Notes on combinations

Given that one can make theoretically convincing cases for many specific combinations, it is reasonable to ask: how good is the evidence that they actually work? A short book such as this cannot comprehensively describe all outcomes of all possible combinations, even if these were available. In fact they are not, since relatively few combinations have been tested rigorously in any case. This approach requires a complex factorial design to determine the optimal ratio of two drugs and to make a valid comparison with the individual components of the preparation.

The United States Food and Drug Administration has stipulated the following stringent requirements for fixed-dose combinations as first-line therapy, which are worth bearing in mind for combinations in general:

i. the combination should be more effective than the sum of its components

ii. the combined product must be at least as safe as its component parts

iii. the risk/benefit ratio should be better than for either component alone.

These are certainly ambitious targets, but they have given added impetus for more careful and detailed studies of this issue. In practice, most studies have included a thiazide or thiazide-like diuretic, so it

> **Relatively few combinations have been tested rigorously**

may be helpful to divide the data broadly into diuretic and non-diuretic studies.[60]

> 66 *It is now generally accepted that the inclusion of diuretics will almost always enhance the efficacy of any combination therapy* 99

### Diuretic-based combinations

The concept of a low or very low dose of diuretic added to another drug has recently attracted even more interest. It is now generally accepted that the inclusion of these drugs will almost always enhance the efficacy of any combination therapy. In the USA the combination of hydrochlorothiazide at a very low dose of just 6.25mg is available in combination with the relatively cardioselective beta-blocker bisoprolol (2.5, 5 and 10mg daily) and has been approved for once-daily dosage in the initial treatment of hypertension. With the 6.25/10 combination, about two-thirds of moderately hypertensive patients have diastolic blood pressures reduced to 90mmHg or less. Although there may be somewhat greater efficacy with 25mg of hydrochlorothiazide, this would certainly be at the expense of more dose-related adverse effects.

Far more combinations involve a thiazide diuretic and an ACE inhibitor. In most publications the thiazide used is hydrochloro-thiazide, typically at a dose of 12.5–25mg, though at higher doses in some of the earlier studies. The ACE inhibitors have included enalapril, perindopril and lisinopril among others. Perindopril has also been widely used in combination with the thiazide-like diuretic indapamide, most notably in the PROGRESS study,[61] where stroke was reduced by about 40% and coronary events by about 28% with combination therapy, which produced a blood pressure reduction of 12/5mmHg. Perindopril on its own did reduce blood pressure by 5/3mmHg but did not significantly reduce the risk of cardiovascular events. Similarly thiazides and AIIRAs constitute a rational and widely used combination.

### Non-diuretic based combinations

Although these combinations are much less common, interest in these has also been increasing recently. In the USA the ACE inhibitor/calcium-channel blocker combination of benazepril and amlodipine has been extensively studied, as part of the development of a combined product.

A combined formulation of trandolapril and verapamil is now available in the UK. A large factorial study with verapamil modified-release (120 or 180mg daily), trandolapril (0.5, 1.0 or 2.0mg daily), and all combinations of these, showed a clear advantage for the combinations. This finding was particularly marked for verapamil 180mg with trandolapril 0.5 or 1.0mg.

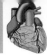

Felodipine and modified-release metoprolol (a relatively cardioselective beta-blocker) have also been studied both individually and in combination. The doses were felodipine 5–10mg daily, metoprolol 50–100mg daily or felodipine plus metoprolol 5/50–10/100mg daily. Blood pressure control, as judged by diastolic 90mmHg or less, was achieved in 45% of patients on felodipine, in 40% of those on metoprolol and in 71% of those taking the combination of the two.

## The efficacy of combinations: an overview

It is very difficult to compare trials of combination therapy, for obvious reasons. There is no overall co-ordination or standardization of trial design but, as for any meta-analysis, some minimum standards for comparability. A remarkable meta-analysis[62] by Law and Wald, and their colleagues (the inventors of the polypill), examines no fewer than 354 randomized clinical trials in hypertension, involving thiazides, beta-blockers, ACE inhibitors, AIIRAs and calcium-channel blockers, and 56,000 patients, of whom 40,000 had been treated with active drugs and the remainder given placebo. In 50 of these trials drugs from two categories were studied separately and in combination, and there were a total of over 100 placebo-controlled comparisons. The authors drew the following conclusions from this huge body of data:

- all five major classes of drug had similar overall efficacy: at full dose an average blood pressure reduction of 9.1/5.5mmHg and a reduction of 7.1/4.4mmHg at half standard dose
- the drugs were effective regardless of baseline levels of blood pressure but, as might be expected, produced greater reductions the higher the initial pressure
- the blood pressure reductions of different classes in combination were additive at either full or half standard doses
- adverse effects, except for ACE inhibitors, were strongly dose related and were essentially undetectable for AIIRAs
- adverse effects were less than additive and serious metabolic problems such as hypokalaemia were negligible at half standard doses of drugs.

It is therefore clear that:

- low-dose combination therapy increases efficacy
- it reduces the likelihood of adverse reactions.

The authors further calculate that in a patient with a starting blood pressure of 150/90mmHg using three drugs at half standard doses (there are actually no trials of three-drug combinations) would reduce pressure by 20/11mmHg and consequently reduce the risk of stroke by 63% and of ischaemic cardiac events by nearly half.

*"It is very difficult to compare trials of combination therapy"*

*"Low dose combination therapy increases efficacy and reduces the likelihood of adverse reactions"*

The question therefore arises:

*Should low-dose combination therapy with two appropriate drugs be the first step in the treatment of essential hypertension?*

Many of us would say that the answer to this is yes, especially if the patient's blood pressure is 20/10mmHg above the target. The ESH/ESC guidelines suggest the plan outlined in Figure 42.

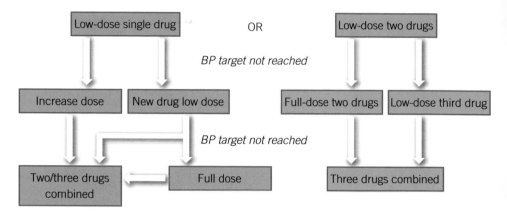

**Fig. 42 Treatment pathway following decision to treat.** Based on current European guidelines.

> *The fixed–dose approach has become more widely acceptable, particularly as regards low–dose combinations*

### Are fixed-dose combinations still controversial?

It is likely that individualized combinations will evolve during the course of the management of individual hypertensive patients, even if they are not used as first-line therapy: as we have seen, most patients will need such combinations for satisfactory control. However, there is still disagreement and controversy about the role of fixed-dose combinations, particularly as a basis for initial therapy. Such combinations have been discouraged in the past, especially in the UK, and particularly by academic clinical pharmacologists! Despite this the fixed-dose approach has become more widely acceptable, particularly as regards low-dose combinations. Recent guidelines, including those of the US Joint National Committee (in both the JNC VI and 7 versions) and the European Society of Hypertension, agree that these preparations are appropriate at least in some circumstances. Obviously, the combination should be a safe and rational one in the first place. The following advantages may follow in addition to those seen with combination therapy in general:

- Reduced numbers of tablets, with potentially improved adherence by patients ("I am taking so many tablets now, doctor" is frequently said and too often true).
- Depending on the national funding system and the manufacturers' pricing structure, reduced costs to the patients, the funding

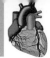

authorities, or both. This certainly seems the likely outcome in the UK.

- The use of doses of drugs that may be lower than those available individually, especially in the case of thiazide diuretics, though there is still considerable progress to be made in this context.

However, there are possible disadvantages that cannot be totally ignored:

- Reduced flexibility in the dosage of individual components.
- Discrepancies in the pharmacokinetics of the component drugs, so that they do not match – usually an avoidable problem in the development of the formulation.
- The danger that prescribers may not always know exactly what the combination contains, especially as regards the contraindications of the individual components.

The first of these issues is undoubtedly a genuine problem. Its effect can be reduced by producing several different combined formulations, but this may be confusing, possibly expensive, and to an extent reduces the usefulness of the basic concept. A simpler approach is to recognize that these preparations should be used only over a narrow dose range, almost always only one or two tablets. It is obviously desirable that chosen doses are based on careful investigations of the possible different combinations, and, as we have seen, this is now increasingly being done. The second issue can be foreseen and avoided by the development and use of appropriate formulations: examples already quoted include extended-release formulations of relatively short-acting drugs such as indapamide and metoprolol, which were combined with intrinsically long-acting drugs (perindopril and felodipine). Not all of these combinations are actually available in the UK, no doubt because of the resistance already mentioned. The third is largely a matter of education: as such it can be minimized but will realistically be impossible to avoid altogether.

> **"Fixed-dose preparations should be used only over a narrow dose range, almost always only one or two tablets"**

### Not just what, but also when?

Blood pressure follows a diurnal rhythm in all people with normal blood pressure and in most hypertensives (Figure 43). Not surprisingly, so does the incidence of cardiovascular events, which shows a marked increase on getting up in the morning associated with rises in blood pressure and heart rate[63] (Figure 44). The control of blood pressure should try to take account of these facts:

- Adequate control should be maintained over the full 24 hours,[64] since there is evidence that less comprehensive control is associated with reduced benefit from treatment. Increased night-time

> **"Blood pressure follows a diurnal rhythm in all people with normal blood pressure and in most hypertensives"**

73

**Fig. 43 The trough-peak ratio.** In this case the ratio of minimal:maximal drug effect is about 50%.

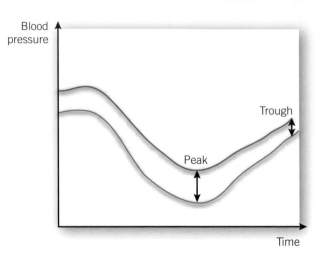

**Fig. 44 Schematic representation of the time distribution of incidence of stroke.** About 30–35% of events occur in the shaded area.

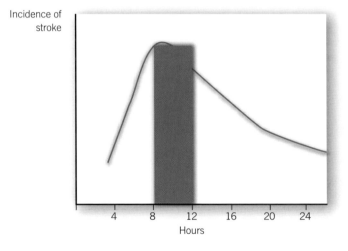

*❝Almost all treatment strategies are directed at once-daily dosing with adequate control throughout the day ❞*

pressures (non-dipping) may be particularly important in increasing the severity of target organ damage.

•   The morning surge in blood pressure should be avoided or minimized.[65]

The first of these objectives has received much greater attention than the second. Almost all treatment strategies are directed at once-daily dosing with adequate control throughout the day, usually characterized by the trough-peak ratio. The US Food and Drug Administration has set a threshold of 0.5 for this ratio if a drug is to be described as a once-daily medication, but most clinicians would regard

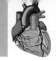

that threshold as inadequate and aim for a value of at least 0.7. The whole concept of the trough-peak ratio has been extensively criticized, but it remains by far the most widely recognized single figure for describing the duration of action of antihypertensive drugs. Alternative approaches, such as the smoothness index, await large-scale validation and general acceptance, though they may have advantages.

The problem of the early morning rise in blood pressure deserves particular emphasis because of the potential clinical consequences. There are three broad approaches:

- changing the formulations
- changing the timing of monotherapy
- using drugs in combination, administered at different times.

The term chronotherapeutics[66] refers to the development of delivery systems that allow drug release not only over an extended period but also at specific times in each 24-hour cycle. This process has been explored in several other therapeutic areas, such as cancer chemotherapy, as well as in hypertension, though it is not very advanced in the latter. Several delivery systems have been developed for the treatment of hypertension, mostly using verapamil as the therapeutic agent, all of which are designed to produce maximum plasma levels of drug between 0600 and 1200 hours. However, these formulations do not seem to have entered clinical practice, though whether for clinical or commercial reasons is unclear, and it is also uncertain whether much development of other formulations is taking place. On the whole this is still a rather neglected area of therapy.

Several studies have compared the efficacy of evening drug administration with the conventional practice of taking the drugs at or after breakfast. There are two potential problems with evening administration. First, blood pressure may drop too much at a time when it is in any case at its lowest, between midnight and 3 am. Though this is unlikely to be noticed by the patient, it could potentially lead to hypoperfusion in already compromised vascular beds, especially in the heart and brain, and possible hypotensive episodes if the patient does get up during the night. Second, and probably more importantly, blood pressure control may be impaired during the late morning and afternoon. Data on this point are contradictory, for instance with discrepant results from the same research group comparing the ACE inhibitors benazepril and quinapril. Overall, it seems unlikely that monotherapy would be a satisfactory solution.

The final and most practicable approach is once again combination therapy. Some drugs (for instance doxazosin) may blunt the morning rise when taken in the evening but by themselves will not provide

> **"***The problem of the early morning rise in blood pressure deserves particular emphasis because of the potential clinical consequences***"**

adequate 24-hour blood pressure control. They can then be combined with other agents, which may be longer acting and would be taken as usual in the morning. It would be rational to use a drug such as doxazosin or a sympatholytic in the evening since they act indirectly or directly on the sympathetic nervous system, which is directly involved in the morning arousal response. In addition, this type of drug can cause sedation, which might be a positive advantage at night but a nuisance during the day. On the negative side, one loses the important advantage of once-daily dosing. It must also be remembered that there is no direct evidence at present for the validity of this approach in terms of reduced morbidity and mortality.

## Special cases

There are several circumstances requiring special consideration in the management of hypertension and some will be discussed here. It is always worth remembering that blood pressure control is always the objective, virtually regardless of precisely how it is achieved.

### The white-coat effect[66]

This has already been mentioned in discussing ABPM and home blood pressure measurements to establish the "true" reading. Usually this is reassuring but in reality the assessment of the overall picture is not so straightforward. The question is essentially the following: how normal is a person who has demonstrated white-coat hypertension? The views on this are very divergent, as is the available data. On balance, but certainly far from unanimously, current opinions suggest that white-coat hypertension is not entirely harmless. Affected individuals may have a cluster of other cardiovascular risk factors and an unknown proportion will develop established hypertension. What then needs to be done? Not surprisingly, there is no consensus, since this has never been properly tested in a prospective clinical trial. It would of course need to be a long trial, probably involving large numbers of subjects: in other words it is unlikely to happen. The new US guidelines might suggest that such people should be regarded as pre-hypertensives (see concluding section) but this is not supported by outcome data and it is not at all clear what one should do in these circumstances. The most realistic advice might be to continue monitoring, at home and occasionally in the surgery or clinic, probably indefinitely.

Recent studies have also revealed the mirror image of this problem, the "reverse white coat" phenomenon.[68] These are patients whose clinic blood pressures are lower than their ambulatory readings. There is obviously a risk that these patients may be undertreated with respect to

> **" Blood pressure control is always the objective, virtually regardless of precisely how it is achieved "**

> **" White-coat hypertension is not entirely harmless "**

their real cardiovascular risk but this needs further investigation particularly in young patients.

### The elderly

By current definitions about two-thirds of this population are hypertensive. The trials of the last decade (e.g. SHEP, Syst-Eur and a significant subset of LIFE)[69–71] have confirmed that treating hypertension in these patients is very rewarding, especially in terms of reduced incidence of stroke, where risk may diminish by as much as 70%. This is not surprising, since it is always those at highest risk who benefit most from interventions. As already noted, these patients are particularly likely to respond to C and D drugs, following the Brown classification discussed earlier, and starting at lower than standard doses may help to minimize side effects, notably postural hypotension. However, they are just as likely to need some form of combination therapy as are younger hypertensives and there is no evidence at all that higher targets should be acceptable. Low-dose combination using the ABCD schema are therefore at least as relevant as in younger patients, and there needs to be particular emphasis on starting at low doses to minimize side effects: the full dose of say amlodipine may be poorly tolerated as initial therapy in a frail 75-year-old patient. There is also evidence for the efficacy of AIIRAs (losartan and candesartan) in reducing adverse outcomes. The treatment of the very elderly (those older than 80 years) will remain debatable at least until the HYVET study is concluded.[72]

### Diabetes and the metabolic syndrome[73]

Aspects of this have already been discussed, with respect to the targets (lower than for non-diabetic patients because of the increased cardio-vascular risk associated with diabetes) and the choice of medication (probably should include an ACE inhibitor or AIIRA). But successful blood pressure lowering is more important than the nature of the drugs that achieve it. In hypertensive patients who are not diabetic but do have the metabolic syndrome there is no reason to think that specific therapies are preferable, though it is arguable that some drugs, notably thiazides and beta-blockers, may accelerate progression of the syndrome. Lifestyle adjustment, with weight loss and increased exercise, is of course critically important for these people. It has been suggested that the thiazolidinediones (pioglitazone and rosiglitazone) may be used in these patients though these drugs may actually promote weight gain even if they lower sugar levels.[74,75] To complicate matters further these drugs may produce small blood pressure reductions by acting as weak calcium-channel blockers but they may also increase the

> **" Treating hypertension in the elderly is very rewarding, especially in terms of reduced incidence of stroke "**

> **" Thiazides and beta-blockers, may accelerate progression of the syndrome "**

> **" Lifestyle adjustment, with weight loss and increased exercise, is critically important "**

*There is a broad consensus that ACE inhibitors or AIIRAs should form part of the treatment regimen*

risk of heart failure or lead to its exacerbation. The current view[76] is that the crucial consideration as far as these hypertensive patients is concerned is efficacy in blood pressure lowering largely irrespective of the actual drugs used. Nevertheless there is a broad consensus that ACE inhibitors or AIIRAs should form part of the treatment regimen.

### Renovascular disease[23,24]

Some of the problems of assessment and management have been mentioned earlier. The medical management involves a paradox: since this is renin-dependent hypertension it is usually responsive, sometimes dramatically and excessively, to ACE inhibitors, and possibly to AIIRAs though the evidence is less clear. Unfortunately, the removal of angiotensin II causes changes in the intrarenal circulation, which will often reduce glomerular filtration rate significantly, perhaps by 50% or even more. In bilateral renal artery disease this can obviously lead to catastrophic decline in kidney function and even to acute, and possibly irreversible, renal failure. It is therefore prudent to avoid these drugs in patients with definite renovascular disease, and to check creatinine levels in all patients within a couple of weeks of starting an ACE inhibitor (probably also an AIIRA), sooner in patients considered high risk. An increase of creatinine of 10% or more is regarded as at least suggestive of renal ischaemia and would encourage withdrawal of the drug. As regards medical treatment in those where revascularization is contraindicated, impossible or refused a combination of other drugs will be required and may be relatively unsuccessful. If so a reconsideration of intervention is of course indicated. This may also help to preserve renal function even if blood pressure is little improved, but even this is debatable.

### Pregnancy[77]

For obvious reasons the management of pregnancy-associated hypertension has made comparatively little progress in relation to other types of hypertension. There are in fact three clinical syndromes included under this heading:

*The management of pregnancy-associated hypertension has made comparatively little progress in relation to other types of hypertension*

- pre-existing hypertension extending into pregnancy
- pregnancy-induced essential hypertension
- pre-eclampsia and eclampsia.

It is certainly not within the scope of this book to discuss the pathogenesis of these conditions, especially of pre-eclampsia, "the disease of hypotheses". Clearly there is not going to be a wealth of clinical trials of antihypertensive medication in this group of patients but the following principles are generally applicable:

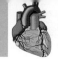

- The definition of hypertension in pregnancy has long been 140/90mmHg, which now approximates to that in the general population. At that level drug treatment is not necessarily indicated though it certainly is at levels >160/110mmHg or, in most specialists' view, >150/100mmHg. In the presence of proteinuria this would certainly be the case.

- Most drugs have not been tested rigorously in pregnant hypertensive patients and some are known to be unsafe, notably ACE inhibitors and AIIRAs.

- The treatments considered to be safe include methyldopa, beta-blockers and labetalol, though there is some evidence of intra-uterine growth retardation in early pregnancy with beta-blockers. Methyldopa has the longest record of safety for both mother and baby and therefore remains the preferred drug of many physicians and obstetricians, although the previously noted side effects are certainly a deterrent for many patients.

- Nifedipine has also been used safely in late pregnancy in severe hypertension. Verapamil also appears to be safe.

- Hydralazine, a vasodilator otherwise little used in hypertension in the UK, is safe and can be effective in severe hypertension including that associated with pregnancy. It may be given orally or intravenously.

- Thiazide diuretics are now considered more favourably than before, provided doses remain low (as they should anyway). They would almost always be used in combination with other agents. However, they may limit the normal plasma volume expansion that occurs in pregnancy and should not be used in situations where this is already a problem, as in pre-eclampsia.

- In severe pre-eclampsia and eclampsia it is recognized that intravenous magnesium sulphate has a unique combination of antihypertensive and anticonvulsant properties.

> *The treatments considered to be safe include methyldopa, beta-blockers and labetalol*

### Resistant hypertension[78]

The working definition of resistant hypertension would now comprise the following: failure to achieve target blood pressures despite adherence to an appropriate combination of three drugs of which one is a thiazide diuretic. The presumption of adherence of course touches on one of the reasons for apparent treatment resistance: the patients are not actually taking the tablets, or are being prescribed the wrong tablets! However, a number of others need to be taken into consideration, notably:

- unrecognized secondary hypertension, including renal disease
- unrecognized salt and fluid overload

> *The presumption of adherence of course touches on one of the reasons for apparent treatment resistance*

- use and abuse of prescription, over the counter or recreational drugs.

There is no single correct approach to this problem but some principles are relevant:

- Consider measurement of plasma renin and adjust medication accordingly (this will usually require withdrawal for 1–2 weeks of drugs directly affecting this hormone, such as beta-blockers. Clearly this may not always be practicable or safe.)
- Consider adding doxazosin to regimen if not already being used.
- Consider adding spironolactone. This has become increasingly widely used in truly resistant cases, though it is far from clear why it works.[79] The efficacy does not seem to be at all related to circulating aldosterone levels. Note that there is considerable risk of hyperkalaemia if this drug is used in combination with an ACE inhibitor or AIIRA: this is not an absolute contraindication but very careful monitoring is required.

Even so, there is a very small minority of patients who are apparently resistant to all medication, no matter how appropriate, and who do adhere to their treatment very closely. The reasons for this are very poorly understood at the moment but almost every practice and clinic will have such patients (thankfully usually only a handful, since they can cause much anxiety!).

> *There is a very small minority of patients who are apparently resistant to all medication*

### Hypertensive emergencies and urgencies[80,81] (Figure 45)

Occasionally, both in primary and secondary care, we are confronted with a patient with extremely high blood pressure. Many will be cared for in intensive care or coronary care units. Although a blood pressure of say 230/130mmHg is certainly alarming it does not necessarily constitute an emergency. From a practical point of view we can regard a hypertensive emergency as high blood pressure (usually >210/130mmHg but possibly lower in pregnancy) associated with acute end-organ damage, including situations that are potentially life-threatening. This includes malignant hypertension where a diastolic pressure of 130mmHg or greater is associated with haemorrhages, exudates and possibly papilloedema, grade III or IV retinal changes according to the conventional classification. Hypertensive urgencies (not a term that is universally accepted in the UK!) are seen in patients with high blood pressure but no immediate evidence of a life-threatening situation or of acute tissue damage. In considering how to manage these patients it is at least as important to avoid certain actions as to perform others. In particular, it is very clear that excessively rapid blood pressure reduction is dangerous and may lead to acute ischaemic

> *Excessively rapid blood pressure reduction is dangerous and may lead to acute ischaemic stroke or myocardial infarction*

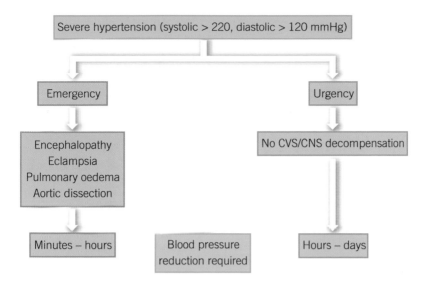

Fig. 45 **Emergency and urgency hypertension.**

stroke or myocardial infarction. Although there is still no definitive consensus, it is generally recommended that:

- Blood pressure is lowered within hours or days rather than minutes.
- The target should not be normalization in the first instance but a diastolic pressure of 100–110mmHg or a 25% reduction in initial mean arterial pressure (remember that mean pressure = diastolic pressure + [pulse pressure/3]) In patients with ischaemic stroke it has been recommended that the diastolic reduction should not exceed 20%, to avoid further aggravating ischaemic damage. In patients with ischaemic stroke and lower blood pressure there is no evidence that active blood pressure reduction improves outcomes.

In urgencies oral therapy is indicated, with the drug of choice probably being a long-acting dihydropyridine, such as modified-release nifedipine or felodipine. The immediately acting capsule formulation of nifedipine must not be used, as it can cause uncontrolled catastrophic falls in blood pressure.

In patients with genuine emergencies, intravenous therapy is preferable but assumes that very close monitoring is available. Sodium nitroprusside is an extremely potent vasodilator with a very short duration of action (seconds). It can therefore be given intravenously with close titration of response, which must be by intra-arterial blood pressure measurement.

Glyceryl trinitrate is an alternative that may be preferred in patients with ischaemic heart disease or where intra-arterial measurements of blood pressure are not available, though this is still preferable. Labetalol, a mixed alpha- and beta-blocker, is also used parenterally in emergencies but response is less predictable and reliable.

Severe hypertension is associated with activation of the renin-angiotensin system, whatever the underlying cause, and addition of a low-dose ACE inhibitor, such as captopril, may be helpful in conjunction with the vasodilators just mentioned. However, there is again the risk of precipitous falls in blood pressure. This can also occur when a beta-blocker is given in conjunction with vasodilators that had further raised renin levels – these are usually elevated in severe hypertension from virtually any cause.

In the specific situation of a dissecting aortic aneurysm the addition of a beta-blocker is important to reduce the force of the systolic pressure wave hitting the aortic wall.

After recovery from the acute phase it is important to remember that emergencies are much more likely in patients with an underlying cause for their hypertension. In patients who present as emergencies, or those previously treated with no known evidence of secondary hypertension, investigation should be reviewed and renewed after recovery.

> *Emergencies are much more likely in patients with an underlying cause for their hypertension*

## Conclusions

Hypertension is more difficult than it looks, as mentioned at the beginning of this book. It is also extremely common and going to become ever more so as populations age in the developed world. It is worth remembering that this is not an inevitable part of human biology: there are a diminishing number of societies where ageing does not lead inevitably to hypertension. However, most of us are working in environments where it almost certainly will. The question of definitions is therefore crucially important. In this context the JNCV7 guidelines, already mentioned on several occasions, are particularly interesting and perhaps even alarming. The concept that individuals with systolic blood pressure greater than 120mmHg are pre-hypertensive can have both negative and beneficial effects. On the one hand, it can hugely increase the number of patients, cause considerable increase in public anxiety and increase the workload of health professionals. On the other, it draws attention to the fact that vascular risk is increased even at these levels and there is the possibility at least that these people may avoid established hypertension in later life by alterations in their lifestyle. The ultimate balance is uncertain, while the other recommendations are less controversial. The current European and even more recent British guidelines have not, however,

> *The concept that individuals with systolic blood pressure greater than 120mmHg are pre-hypertensive can have both negative and beneficial effects*

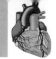

adopted the concept of prehypertension and agree on the definitions described in Figure 5.

Another issue that needs consideration is the relationship between hypertension and global cardiovascular risk. In deciding whether to prescribe statins, it is usual to estimate the overall risk by means of charts or computer-based algorithms. In practice it is the blood pressure figures alone that matter when deciding to initiate treatment for hypertension. However, there are grey areas such as patients with systolic blood pressure in the 140–150mmHg range without target organ damage, where risk assessment may make a significant difference to decisions concerning intervention. The general message must again be always to take into account the overall cardiovascular risk status of the patient.

Another question that most of us will have pondered concerns new drugs in hypertension: do we need them and are we going to get some that are really more effective than those we have today? A colleague commented recently that it made a welcome change to use drugs like the statins, which actually worked, as opposed to antihypertensive drugs, which did not. Rather a harsh judgement perhaps but certainly the statins can lower cholesterol by 50–60% while antihypertensives on average are likely to manage 10–15% reductions in pressure as monotherapy. In some ways this may not be such a disadvantage, since we have seen on a number of occasions that excessive blood pressure lowering, at least if it is done quickly, is potentially dangerous. Are we going to get a "super pill" for hypertension? It is not very likely: the vasopeptidase inhibitors, which showed promise as having slightly greater efficacy especially in reducing systolic blood pressure, appear to cause angioedema too frequently to be used as first-line drugs though some sort of reserve role in resistant patients may still be feasible. The "polypill" proposed by Law and Wald[82] is a combination of six existing drugs including three antihypertensive agents – a topic for another discussion but this author is not an enthusiast! The Anglo-Scandinavian Cardiovascular Outcomes Trial (ASCOT),[83] involving over 19,000 patients will be reporting by 2005 and is likely to be the last large-scale attempt to establish in a clinical trial whether any particular class of drug is clearly better in terms of real clinical end-points. Even if it cannot answer that question (to which there may be no unequivocal answer) it should still provide a mass of useful information about the drugs we use.

Meanwhile, The Blood Pressure Lowering Treatments Trialists Collaboration (BPLTTC) have now analysed 29 trials involving over 160,000 patients and concluded that:[84,85]

> **"It is the blood pressure figures alone that matter when deciding to initiate treatment for hypertension"**

> **"Antihypertensives on average are likely to manage 10–15% reductions in pressure as monotherapy"**

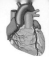

> *In a large clinic population outcomes with ACE inhibitors were found to be significantly better than those with calcium–channel blockers*

- ACE inhibitors, calcium-channel blockers, diuretics and beta-blockers had similar effects on reducing the risk of cardiovascular events, as did AIIRAs
- there may be small advantages for specific drugs for specific outcomes: diuretics and calcium-channel blockers may have greater effects on stroke, while ACE inhibitors, and perhaps AIIRAs, may have greater efficacy in the prevention of heart failure
- the greater the reduction in blood pressure the fewer strokes and other events, with the possible exception of heart failure
- magnitude of blood pressure reduction was more important than the choice of drug.

It has to be noted that there are dissenting views on the last point: for instance, in a large clinic population outcomes with ACE inhibitors were found to be significantly better than those with calcium-channel blockers.[86]

Some concluding suggestions are summarized in Figure 46.

Fig. 46 A summary of the management of primary hypertension.

---

**A summary of the management of primary hypertension**

- Non-pharmacological approaches should be used if appropriate but should not delay the introduction of drug therapy if indicated
- The main classes of antihypertensive drugs are all effective
- Initial choice of therapy should be individualized as far as possible
- Low-dose combination therapy should be considered at the outset, especially if blood pressure is 20/10 mmHg or more above target levels
- The target blood pressure should be less than 140/85 mmHg in general but less than 130/80 mmHg in patients with diabetes, renal disease or existing cardiovascular disease
- If blood pressure is well controlled six-monthly follow-up is usually adequate

---

But, even if we do not have "perfect" treatments for hypertension, let us not lose sight of the fact that we are still very much luckier than our clinical predecessors. A few years ago the *BMJ* printed the blood pressure graph for the late President Franklin D Roosevelt in the last months of his life. The inexorable rise to systolic pressures of 300mmHg or more was totally beyond the control of his physicians. That is a situation we should not have to face.

All the case histories below are based on real histories. Of course they represent only a tiny sample of the possible clinical scenarios but one hopes they contain some useful pointers on management. There are few dogmatic rules in hypertension (at least not ones that happen to be correct!) and the reader may well take a different approach.

## Case study 1

### The metabolic syndrome and Type 2 diabetes

Mr C is the 57-year-old regional manager of a company supplying spare parts to garages. He is completely asymptomatic. He undergoes a medical examination for life insurance. His blood pressure is found to be 154/106mmHg (confirmed on two more occasions). His weight is 96kg and his BMI is 32 with a waist circumference of 104cm: he is very fond of pasta! Urinalysis was positive for protein. Apart from some arteriolar narrowing in the fundi (Grade I), there was nothing else of note on examination. He takes little or no exercise, has never smoked, and drinks 1–2 glasses of wine a day. The results of relevant investigations are summarized below.

*66 His weight is 96kg and his BMI is 32 with a waist circumference of 104cm 99*

| Investigation | Result (reference range) |
|---|---|
| Plasma potassium | 4.2mmol/l (3.5–5) |
| Serum creatinine | 112mmol/l (<130) |
| Fasting glucose | 7.6mmol/l (<5.4) |
| HbA$_{1c}$ | 8.4%   (<6.0) |
| Serum total cholesterol | 4.8mmol/l (<5.0) |
| LDL cholesterol | uncertain because of high triglycerides |
| HDL cholesterol | 0.71mmol/l (>1.0) |
| Total cholesterol:HDL ratio | see above |
| Triglycerides | 17.2mmol/l (<2.0) |
| Renal ultrasound | Normal |

*66 Mr C clearly has the features of the metabolic syndrome 99*

## Comment and management

Mr C clearly has the features of the metabolic syndrome: central obesity, Type 2 diabetes, dyslipidaemia and, of course, hypertension. All of the above need therapeutic intervention:

• Advice on weight reduction, diet and increased exercise and explanation of the risks of the existing situation.

> *These very high levels of serum triglycerides predispose to acute pancreatitis*

- Control of dyslipidaemia, preferably with a fibrate (fenofibrate in this instance). Note that these very high levels of serum triglycerides predispose to acute pancreatitis if they are not promptly lowered.
- Control of hyperglycamia with diet combined with an oral hypo-glycaemic agent. Metformin is the first choice since it tends to decrease appetite and weight. In the absence of renal, hepatic or cardiac impairment, as in this case, the risk of lactic acidosis is extremely small. There is some evidence that metformin can delay the appearance of overt diabetes during the phase of glucose intolerance but is less effective than lifestyle modification.
- Control of hypertension. In the presence of diabetes, ACE inhibitors or angiotensin II receptor antagonists are almost always used as part of the treatment regimen. He was started on perindopril, which was well tolerated but did not by itself reduce blood pressure to target levels: 130/80mmHg in view of the concurrent diabetes.

## Progress

Blood pressure proved very easy to control on a combination of perindopril (4mg daily) and amlodipine (5mg daily). Pressures of 115–120/70–80mmHg were achieved and maintained within 2 months. However, hyperglycaemia was poorly controlled on metformin alone (2g daily) with a $HbA_{1c}$ of 7.2%, and he is being considered for thiazolidinedione therapy by the Diabetes Clinic. His triglycerides fell to 5.2mmol/l but have since risen again to 8.3mmol/l while his HDL is very low at 0.43mmol/l (all while on fenofibrate 267mg daily). He was not able to tolerate a statin because of myalgia and is starting therapy with nicotinic acid and high-dose omega-3 fatty acids in addition to the fibrate. He has failed to lose any weight.

> *Blood pressure proved very easy to control*

In this instance blood pressure has proved the easiest abnormality to correct, despite the lack of success with the metabolic problems. Often blood pressure remains "resistant" in these circumstances, so that triple or quadruple antihypertensive therapy is needed. If so, a low-dose thiazide, preferably indapamide, should almost always form part of the combination. Readers will not need reminding that weight targets can be extremely difficult to attain or even approach.

> *Weight targets can be extremely difficult to attain*

- Look for other elements of the metabolic syndrome in all hypertensive patients
- Management of all risk factors should be carried out in parallel

## Case study 2

### Isolated systolic hypertension

Mrs M is an exceptionally active 83-year-old lady. She is fully independent and recently visited her son in Australia. An annual check-up carried out by her general practitioner was entirely reassuring except for her blood pressure, which was 192/76mmHg on average after repeated measurements. Physical examination was otherwise normal. Relevant examinations are summarized below.

*66 An annual check–up carried out by her general practitioner was entirely reassuring except for her blood pressure 99*

| Investigation | Result |
|---|---|
| Plasma potassium | 4.1mmol/l |
| Serum creatinine | 122mmol/l |
| Fasting blood glucose | 5.0mmol/l |
| ECG | Normal (minor T wave changes) |
| Echocardiogram | Increased left ventricular mass index and septal wall thickness (moderate hypertrophy) |
| Renal ultrasound | Normal |

## Comment and management

This lady has isolated systolic hypertension but is otherwise entirely well. However, she does have a moderate degree of left ventricular hypertrophy and clinical trials strongly support treatment in this situation, especially to reduce the risk of stroke. A low-dose thiazide, bendroflumethiazide (bendrofluazide) 2.5mg daily, would be rational evidence-based treatment.

*66 Clinical trials strongly support treatment in this situation 99*

## Progress

After 6 weeks of therapy, blood pressure had fallen to 176/74mmHg with no side effects. Perindopril 4mg daily was added with a good response but a persistent dry cough, so irbesartan 75mg then 150mg daily was substituted for perindopril. This was preferred to say losartan or candesartan because of the age-related impairment in renal function and the dual mode of clearance of this drug. After 2 months of combination therapy blood pressure was 148/72mmHg. Mrs M was reluctant to increase her medication further, though strictly speaking her systolic pressures were above target. She remains well and free of side effects.

Low-dose long-acting dihydropyridines (felodipine or amlodipine) are also
alternative first-line therapy in a patient like this. Note that as always
treatment is a matter of negotiation: not all our patients may share our
enthusiasm for targets!

- Thiazides or long-acting dihydropyridines are good first-line treatment in
  isolated systolic hypertension but are usually not sufficient as monotherapy

## Case study 3

### Borderline hypertension

Mr B is a 31-year-old man taking a law conversion course. His father, a
retired consultant physician, suggested that his general practitioner
should refer him for further investigations after a series of blood pressure
readings in the surgery of 140–145/90–95mmHg with a resting pulse
of about 80/minute. Mr B is physically well but is sleeping poorly and is
anxious about his future career. He has never smoked and drinks wine
socially and spirits rarely. His BMI is 26 and there is nothing of note
on examination apart from the blood pressure and pulse. His mother
developed hypertension in her 60s. Investigations are summarized below.

| Investigation | Result |
|---|---|
| Serum potassium | 4.4mmol/l |
| Serum creatinine | 89mmol/l |
| Serum total cholesterol | 4.2mmol/l |
| HDL cholesterol | 1.8mmol/l |
| Fasting blood glucose | 4.9mmol/l |
| ECG | Normal |
| Echocardiogram | Normal |
| Renal ultrasound | Normal |
| 24 hour ABPM | Daytime mean 129/82mmHg |
| | Night-time mean 120/81mmHg |

## Comment and management

There is no evidence of target organ damage or of any other cardiovascular risk factors. On ambulatory blood pressure monitoring his mean
daytime pressure is just within the normal range and there is a nocturnal
dip that is slightly less than predicted. It is not at all clear what if
anything needs to be done here, since the evidence does not exist.

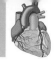

Options include:

1. Treating with a centrally acting sympatholytic drug, probably moxonidine.
2. Recommending lifestyle changes and other measures such as relaxation therapies where relevant and continuing follow-up once or twice a year.
3. Some combination of 1 and 2.

Most clinicians will probably choose the second option, but whether or not this influences outcomes is unknown. Although beta-blockers might seem an obvious choice, in fact they have not proved useful in curbing the white-coat response. They may still, of course, reduce tachycardia and other physical symptoms of anxiety other than the rise in blood pressure.

- **Borderline hypertension, often with a white-coat effect, has no clearly defined therapy beyond extended follow-up**

## Case study 4

### "Ordinary" hypertension

Mrs D is a 54-year-old lady who consulted her general practitioner because of occasional morning headaches. At the surgery her blood pressure on several occasions was 162/104mmHg, with Grade I fundal changes but no other abnormalities on examination other than a BMI of 26 (weight 72kg). She has two grown-up children and had mildly elevated blood pressure but not pre-eclampsia during both pregnancies. Her blood pressure had returned to normal levels after each delivery and had been measured very infrequently for the past 20 years. She had given up smoking 3 years earlier and drank a couple of glasses of wine a day. She took multivitamin pills but no other medication. Investigations are shown below.

> *Mildly elevated blood pressure but not pre-eclampsia during both pregnancies*

| Investigation | Result (reference range) |
| --- | --- |
| Serum potassium | 3.9mmol/l |
| Serum creatinine | 101mmol/l |
| Fasting blood glucose | 5.1mmol/l |
| Serum total cholesterol | 4.8mmol/l |
| HDL cholesterol | 1.6mmol/l |
| LDL cholesterol | 2.6mmol/l (<2.6) |
| Total cholesterol:HDL ratio | 3.0 (<5.0) |
| ECG | Normal |
| Echocardiogram | Mild/moderate hypertrophy |

*" There is no clear first choice for first–line medication "*

## Comment and management

This lady has moderate (Grade 2 – not to be confused with the retinal grades) hypertension with evidence of retinal change and in particular left ventricular hypertrophy. Her hypertension should be treated, but at this age and with relative absence of other risk factors there is no clear first choice for first-line medication. It would be reasonable to use a fixed low-dose combination, and she was treated with irbesartan 150mg/hydrochlorothiazide 12.5mg daily. She was also given dietary advice to promote weight loss of about 5–6kg.

## Progress

Renal function was checked after 1 week in case there was unsuspected renovascular disease, but creatinine had risen by only 3mmol/l. At that time blood pressure was 152/96mmHg and she had experienced only one mild headache. The same medication was continued and she was reviewed again 4 weeks later. At this time she had lost 3kg in weight and her blood pressure was 145/92mmHg. She was prescribed doxazosin 4mg at night and 1 month later her blood pressure was 136/85mmHg and she was asymptomatic. She had lost a further 1kg in weight.

*" Most "ordinary" hypertension will also need combination therapy "*

- Most "ordinary" hypertension will also need combination therapy
- Fixed-dose combinations are useful parts of combination therapy
- Pre-eclampsia or other transient hypertension during pregnancy increases the risk of sustained hypertension in later life

### Case study 5

#### Primary hyperaldosteronism

Mr W is a 58-year-old bank manager who saw his general practitioner because of headaches and malaise. His blood pressure then was consistently about 170/110mmHg. There were Grade II changes in the fundi and an ECG showed left ventricular hypertrophy. Serum creatinine and electrolytes were recorded as normal. He was treated with a variety of drugs including calcium-channel blockers, beta-blockers, ACE inhibitors and thiazides. The latter were discontinued because potassium levels fell to 3.1mmol/l. The drugs alone and in various combinations failed to reduce blood pressure by more than 15/10mmHg. He was

*" The drugs alone and in various combinations failed to reduce blood pressure by more than 15/10mmHg "*

| Investigation | Result (reference range) |
|---|---|
| Serum potassium | 3.6mmol/l |
| Serum creatinine | 118mmol/l |
| Plasma renin | < 0.2mmol/l (usually > 0.3) |
| Plasma aldosterone:renin ratio | 1800 (<1000) |
| ECG | Left ventricular hypertrophy |
| Echocardiogram | Moderate/severe hypertrophy |

*66 There is clear evidence for an inappropriately high plasma aldosterone level 99*

referred for further assessment after having stopped all medication at his own request. His initial investigations, after 3 weeks off all medication, are summarized above.

## Comment and management

There is clear evidence for an inappropriately high plasma aldosterone level in this patient, though his plasma potassium is still within the normal range. Note that he was highly sensitive to thiazide-induced hypokalaemia. CT scans of the adrenals revealed bilateral enlargement. He was treated with 12.5mg spironolactone twice a day increasing after a week to 25mg twice daily. At the same time he was given amlodipine 5mg daily. In the light of bilateral disease, surgery was not a realistic option and the patient indicated that he would have refused it even for unilateral disease.

## Progress

After 6 weeks the blood pressure on the above regimen had fallen to 148/93mmHg and the serum potassium was 4.5mmol/l. He felt well apart from slight bilateral gynaecomastia. On increasing the dose of amlodipine to 10mg daily the blood pressure fell after a month to 137/86mmHg, with minimal ankle oedema.

*66 Some patients require higher doses of spironolactone or addition of amiloride 99*

Note that this was a relatively easy case to manage: some patients require higher doses of spironolactone or addition of amiloride to correct the hypokalaemia as well as control the blood pressure.

- Patients with primary hyperaldosteronism may have normal plasma potassium levels but readily become hypokalaemic when given a thiazide
- Patients with primary hyperaldosteronism may have severe hypertension that is very resistant to treatment unless spironolactone is included

66 *She complained of tiredness for several months, without other specific symptoms* 99

### Hypertension in an Afro-Caribbean patient

Ms P is a 47-year-old secretary working in a general practice surgery. Her family was originally from Jamaica and her mother and two sisters were being treated for high blood pressure: her mother had suffered a small stroke from which she had made a full recovery. She complained of tiredness for several months, without other specific symptoms, and consulted her own general practitioner. He noted a blood pressure of 184/110mmHg on repeated measurement, with Grade II fundal changes and a thrusting and displaced left ventricular apex beat. Urinalysis was positive for protein. ECG showed undoubted left ventricular hypertrophy and other investigations are shown below.

66 *This lady has primary hypertension with very much suppressed plasma renin activity, as is often the case with black hypertensive patients* 99

| Investigation | Result |
|---|---|
| Serum potassium | 4.6mmol/l |
| Serum creatinine | 139mmol/l |
| Plasma renin activity | <0.2mmol/l |
| Plasma aldosterone:renin ratio | 520 |
| Echocardiogram | Severe hypertrophy |

## Comment and management

This lady has primary hypertension with very much suppressed plasma renin activity, as is often the case with black hypertensive patients. She has creatinine slightly higher than the reference range and this reflects renal impairment, which is also often disproportionate in this group of patients. She is not diabetic, though this too is often a common concurrent problem. She was started on a triple combination of amlodipine 5mg daily and fixed combination irbesartan 150mg/hydrochlorothiazide 12.5mg daily.

## Progress

Ms P's blood pressure after a month of the above regimen had fallen to 161/98mmHg. At this point her creatinine had decreased slightly to 126mmol/l. The amlodipine was increased to 10mg daily and the fixed combination to the higher strength containing irbesartan 300mg/hydrochlorothiazide 12.5mg daily. Blood pressure after a further 4 weeks was 146/88mmHg. Her creatinine remained stable.

66 *Black hypertensives (from the Caribbean and the USA especially) often have severe hypertension needing multiple drugs* 99

- Black hypertensives (from the Caribbean and the USA especially) often have severe hypertension needing multiple drugs accompanied by left ventricular hypertrophy and early renal impairment

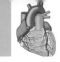

## Thiazide diuretics

| Drug | Trade name | Preparation | Strength | Doses used in hypertension (adult) | Comments | Side effects |
|---|---|---|---|---|---|---|
| Bendroflu-methiazide (bendrofluazide) | Generic | Tablet | 2.5, 5 mg | 2.5 mg mane | Drug of choice for elderly patients; contraindicated in patients with gout; caution in hepatic and renal impairment, pregnancy and breast feeding | Postural hypotension, mild gastrointestinal effects, impotence, hypokalaemia, hypomagnesaemia, hyponatraemia, hypocalcaemia, hypochloraemic alkalosis, hyperuricaemia, gout, hyperglycaemia, altered plasma lipid concentrations |
| Bendroflu-methiazide + potassium | Centyl K | Tablet | 2.5 mg + 7.7 mmol | 1 tablet mane | Combination of thiazide and potassium-sparing diuretics preferable; swallow whole with plenty of water | |
| | Neo-NaClex-K | Tablet | 2.5 mg + 8.4 mmol | 1 tablet mane | | |
| Chlortalidone (chlorthalidone) | Hygroton | Tablet | 50 mg | 25 mg mane increasing to 50 mg prn | Drug of choice for elderly patients; contraindicated in patients with gout; caution in hepatic and renal impairment, pregnancy and breast feeding | Postural hypotension, mild gastrointestinal effects, impotence, hypokalaemia, hypomagnesaemia, hyponatraemia, hypocalcaemia, hypochloraemic alkalosis, hyperuricaemia, gout, hyperglycaemia, altered plasma lipid concentrations |
| Cyclopen-thiazide | Navidrex | Tablet | 500 mcg | 250 mcg mane increasing to 500 mcg prn | Drug of choice for elderly patients; contraindicated in patients with gout; use with other drugs if hypertension is not controlled with low dose | Postural hypotension, mild gastrointestinal effects, impotence, hypokalaemia, hypomagnesaemia, hyponatraemia, hypocalcaemia, hypochloraemic alkalosis, hyperuricaemia, gout, hyperglycaemia, altered plasma lipid concentrations |

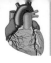

## Thiazide diuretics

| Drug | Trade name | Preparation | Strength | Doses used in hypertension (adult) | Comments | Side effects |
|---|---|---|---|---|---|---|
| Hydrochloro-thiazide | | | | | Contraindicated in patients with gout; caution in hepatic and renal impairment, pregnancy and breast feeding | Postural hypotension, mild gastrointestinal effects, impotence, hypokalaemia, hypomagnesaemia, hyponatraemia, hypocalcaemia, hypochloraemic alkalosis, hyperuricaemia, gout, hyperglycaemia, altered plasma lipid concentrations |
| Indapamide | Natrilix | Tablet | 2.5 mg | 2.5 mg mane | Drug of choice for elderly patients; contraindicated in patients with gout; caution in hepatic and renal impairment, pregnancy and breast feeding | Hypokalaemia, headache, dizziness, fatigue, muscle cramps, nausea, anorexia, diarrhoea, constipation, rashes |
| | Natrilix SR | M/R tablet | 1.5 mg | 1.5 mg mane | | |
| Metolazone | Metenix 5 | Tablet | 5 mg | 5 mg mane; maintenance 5 mg on alternate days | Drug of choice for elderly patients; contraindicated in patients with gout; caution in hepatic and renal impairment, pregnancy and breast feeding | Postural hypotension, mild gastrointestinal effects, impotence, hypokalaemia, hypomagnesaemia, hyponatraemia, hypocalcaemia, hypochloraemic alkalosis, hyperuricaemia, gout, hyperglycaemia, altered plasma lipid concentrations |
| Xipamide | Diurexan | Tablet | 20 mg | 20 mg mane | Drug of choice for elderly patients; contraindicated in patients with gout; caution in hepatic and renal impairment, pregnancy and breast feeding | Gastrointestinal effects, mild dizziness, hypokalaemia and other electrolyte disturbances |

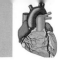

## Loop diuretics

| Drug | Trade name | Preparation | Strength | Doses used in hypertension (adult) | Comments | Side effects |
|------|-----------|-------------|----------|-----------------------------------|----------|--------------|
| Furosemide (frusemide) | Lasix | Tablet | 20, 40, 500 mg | 20–40 mg mane | Used to lower blood pressure in patients with chronic renal failure who have not responded to thiazide diuretics; caution in pregnancy and breast feeding | Hyponatraemia, hypokalaemia, hypomagnesaemia, hypochloraemic alkalosis, increased calcium excretion |
| Bumetanide | Burinex | Tablet | 1, 5 mg | 1 mg mane | Used to lower blood pressure in patients with chronic renal failure who have not responded to thiazide diuretics; caution in pregnancy and breast feeding | Hyponatraemia, hypokalaemia, hypomagnesaemia, hypochloraemic alkalosis, increased calcium excretion, myalgia |
| Torasemide | Torem | Tablet | 2.5, 5, 10 mg | 2.5 mg mane increasing to 5 mg prn | Used to lower blood pressure in patients with chronic renal failure who have not responded to thiazide diuretics; caution in pregnancy and breast feeding | Hyponatraemia, hypokalaemia, hypomagnesaemia, hypochloraemic alkalosis, increased calcium excretion, dry mouth |

## Potassium-sparing diuretics (with other diuretics)

| Drug | Trade name | Preparation | Strength | Doses used in hypertension (adult) | Comments | Side effects |
|------|-----------|-------------|----------|-----------------------------------|----------|--------------|
| Amiloride | Generic | Tablet | 5 mg | 5–10 mg mane | Used in combination with thiazide diuretics to treat hypertension; contraindicated in renal failure; caution in diabetes mellitus, pregnancy and breast feeding | Gastrointestinal effects, dry mouth, rashes, confusion, postural hypotension, hyperkalaemia, hyponatraemia |
| Amiloride + cyclopenthiazide | Navispare | Tablet | 2.5 mg + 250 mcg | 1–2 tablets mane | | See also cyclopenthiazide |
| Amiloride + hydrochloro-thiazide (co-amilozide) | Generic | Tablet | 2.5 + 25, 5 + 50 mg | 2.5 + 25–5 + 50 mg mane (max 5 + 50 mane) | | See also hydrochlorothiazide |

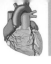

| Potassium-sparing diuretics (with other diuretics) | | | | | |
|---|---|---|---|---|---|
| Drug | Trade name | Preparation | Strength | Doses used in hypertension (adult) | Comments | Side effects |
| Spironolactone | Aldactone | Tablet | 25, 50, 100 mg | 100–200 mg daily increased to 400 mg prn | Potentiates thiazide or loop diuretics; used in Conn's syndrome; contraindicated in hyperkalaemia, hyponatraemia, pregnancy and breast feeding, Addison's disease; caution in hepatic and renal impairment, elderly, porphyria, monitor electrolytes | Gastrointestinal disturbances, impotence, gynaecomastia, menstrual irregularities, lethargy, headache, confusion, rashes, hyperkalaemia, hyponatraemia, hepatotoxicity, osteomalacia, blood disorders |
| Triamterene | Dytac | Capsule | 50 mg | 150–250 mg daily (less with thiazide diuretics), maintenance 150–250 mg on alternate days | Used in combination with thiazide diuretics to treat hypertension; contraindicated in renal failure; caution in diabetes mellitus, pregnancy and breast feeding; take with or after food | Gastrointestinal effects, dry mouth, rashes, hyperkalaemia, hyponatraemia |
| Triamterene + hydrochloro-thiazide (co-triamterzide) | Dyazide | Tablet | 50 + 25 mg | 1 tablet mane (max 4 tablets/day) | | See also hydrochlorothiazide |
| Triamterene + chlortalidone | Kalspare | Tablet | 50 + 50 mg | 1–2 tablets mane | | See also chlortalidone |

| Beta-adrenoceptor blocking drugs | | | | | |
|---|---|---|---|---|---|
| Acebutolol | Sectral | Capsule Tablet | 100, 200, 400 mg | 400 mg/day increasing to 400 mg 2 times/day prn | Contraindicated in asthma, chronic obstructive pulmonary disease and heart block; caution in renal and hepatic impairment, pregnancy and breast feeding | Bradycardia (less likely), heart failure, conduction disorders, bronchospasm, peripheral vasoconstriction (less likely), gastrointestinal effects, fatigue, sleep disturbance |
| Acebutolol + hydrochloro-thiazide | Secadrex | Tablet | 200 + 12.5 mg | 1–2 tablets mane | | See also hydrochlorothiazide |

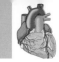

## Beta-adrenoceptor blocking drugs

| Drug | Trade name | Preparation | Strength | Doses used in hypertension (adult) | Comments | Side effects |
|---|---|---|---|---|---|---|
| Atenolol | Tenormin 25 | Tablet | 25 mg | 50 mg/day | Contraindicated in asthma, chronic obstructive pulmonary disease and heart block; accumulates in renal impairment (reduce dose); caution in hepatic impairment, pregnancy and breast feeding | Bradycardia, heart failure, conduction disorders, bronchospasm, peripheral vasoconstriction, gastrointestinal effects, fatigue, sleep disturbance (less likely) |
| | Tenormin LS | Tablet | 50 mg | | | |
| | Tenormin | Tablet | 100 mg | | | |
| Atenolol + bendroflu-methiazide | Tenben | Capsule | 25 + 1.25 mg | 25 + 1.25 mg mane | | See also bendroflumethiazide |
| Atenolol + chlortalidone (co-tenidone) | Tenoret 50 | Tablet | 50 + 12.5 mg | 50 + 12.5-100 + 25 mg mane | | See also chlortalidone |
| | Tenoretic | Tablet | 100 + 25 mg | | | |
| Atenolol + amiloride + hydrochloro-thiazide | Kalten | Capsule | 50 + 2.5 + 25 mg | 1 capsule mane | | See also amiloride and hydrochlorothiazide |
| Atenolol + nifedipine | Beta-Adalat | M/R capsule | 50 + 20 mg | 1-2 capsules/day (elderly 1 capsule/day) | Only indicated when calcium-channel blocker or beta-blocker alone is inadequate; swallow whole | See also nifedipine |
| | Tenif | M/R capsule | 50 + 20 mg | 1-2 capsules/day (elderly 1 capsule/day) | | |
| Betaxolol | Kerlone | Tablet | 20 mg | 20-40 mg/day (elderly 10 mg/day) | Contraindicated in asthma, chronic obstructive pulmonary disease and heart block; relatively cardioselective; accumulates in renal impairment (reduce dose); caution in hepatic impairment, pregnancy and breast feeding | Bradycardia, heart failure, conduction disorders, bronchospasm, peripheral vasoconstriction, gastrointestinal effects, fatigue, sleep disturbance |

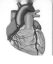

## Beta-adrenoceptor blocking drugs

| Drug | Trade name | Preparation | Strength | Doses used in hypertension (adult) | Comments | Side effects |
|---|---|---|---|---|---|---|
| Bisoprolol | Cardicor | Tablet | 1.25, 2.5, 3.75 5, 7.5, 10 mg | 5–10 mg/day (max 20 mg/day) | Contraindicated in asthma, chronic obstructive pulmonary disease and heart block; relatively cardioselective; accumulates in hepatic and renal impairment (reduce dose); caution in pregnancy and breast feeding | Bradycardia, heart failure, conduction disorders, bronchospasm, peripheral vasoconstriction, gastrointestinal effects, fatigue, sleep disturbance |
| | Emcor | Tablet | 5, 10 mg | | | |
| | Monocor | Tablet | 5, 10 mg | | | |
| Bisoprolol + hydrochloro-thiazide | Monozide 10 | Tablet | 10 + 6.25 mg | 1 tablet/day | | See also hydrochlorothiazide |
| Carvedilol | Eucardic | Tablet | 3.125, 6.25, 12.5, 25 mg | 12.5–25 mg/day (elderly 12.5 mg/day) (max 50 mg/day) | Contraindicated in asthma, chronic obstructive pulmonary disease, heart block and hepatic impairment; caution in renal impairment, pregnancy and breast feeding | Postural hypotension, dizziness, headache, fatigue, gastrointestinal effects, bradycardia |
| Celiprolol | Celectol | Tablet | 200, 400 mg | 200 mg mane increasing to 400 mg prn | Contraindicated in asthma, chronic obstructive pulmonary disease and heart block; accumulates in renal impairment (reduce dose); caution in hepatic impairment, pregnancy and breast feeding; take before food | Headache, dizziness, fatigue, nausea, somnolence |
| Labetolol | Trandate | Tablet | 50, 100, 200, 400 mg | 100–200 mg 2 times/day (elderly 50 mg 2 times/day initially) (max 2.4 g/day) | Contraindicated in asthma, chronic obstructive pulmonary disease, heart block and hepatic impairment; caution in renal impairment, pregnancy and breast feeding; take with or after food | Postural hypotension, tiredness, weakness, headache, rashes, scalp tingling, difficulty in micturition, epigastric pain, nausea, vomiting, liver damage |

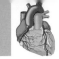

## Beta-adrenoceptor blocking drugs

| Drug | Trade name | Preparation | Strength | Doses used in hypertension (adult) | Comments | Side effects |
|---|---|---|---|---|---|---|
| Metoprolol | Betaloc | Tablet | 50, 100 mg | 100 mg/day; maintenance 100–200 mg/day | Contraindicated in asthma, chronic obstructive pulmonary disease, heart block; accumulates in hepatic impairment (reduce dose); caution in hepatic impairment, pregnancy and breast feeding; M/R formulations should be swallowed whole | Bradycardia, heart failure, conduction disorders, bronchospasm, peripheral vasoconstriction, gastrointestinal effects, fatigue, sleep disturbance |
| | Betaloc-SA | M/R tablet | 200 mg | | | |
| | Lopresor | Tablet | 50, 100 mg | | | |
| | Lopresor SR | M/R tablet | 200 mg | 1 tablet/day | | |
| Metoprolol + hydrochloro-thiazide | Co-Betaloc | Tablet | 100 + 12.5 mg | 1–3 tablets/day | | See also hydrochlorothiazide |
| | Co-Betaloc SA | M/R tablet | 200 + 25 mg | 1 tablet/day | | |
| Nadolol | Corgard | Tablet | 40, 80 mg | 80 mg/day (max 240 mg/day) | Contraindicated in asthma, chronic obstructive pulmonary disease and heart block; caution in renal and hepatic impairment, pregnancy and breast feeding | Bradycardia, heart failure, conduction disorders, bronchospasm, peripheral vasoconstriction, gastrointestinal effects, fatigue, sleep disturbance (less likely) |
| Nadolol + bendroflu-methiazide | Corgaretic | Tablet | 40 + 5, 80 + 5 mg | 1–2 tablets/day | | See also bendroflumethiazide |
| Nebivolol | Nebilet | Tablet | 5 mg | 5 mg/day (elderly 2.5 mg/day initially) | Contraindicated in asthma, chronic obstructive pulmonary disease, heart block and hepatic impairment; accumulates in renal impairment (reduce dose); caution in pregnancy and breast feeding | Bradycardia, heart failure, conduction disorders, bronchospasm, peripheral vasoconstriction, gastrointestinal effects, fatigue, sleep disturbance, oedema, headache, depression, visual disturbances, impotence |

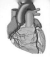

## Beta-adrenoceptor blocking drugs

| Drug | Trade name | Preparation | Strength | Doses used in hypertension (adult) | Comments | Side effects |
|---|---|---|---|---|---|---|
| Oxprenolol | Trasicor | Tablet | 20, 40, 80 mg | 80–160 mg/day in 2–3 divided doses (max 320 mg) | Contraindicated in asthma, chronic obstructive pulmonary disease and heart block; caution in renal and hepatic impairment, pregnancy and breast feeding; M/R formulation should be swallowed whole | Bradycardia (less likely), heart failure, conduction disorders, bronchospasm, peripheral vasoconstriction (less likely), gastrointestinal effects, fatigue, sleep disturbance |
| | Slow-Trasicor | M/R tablet | 160 mg | 160 mg/day (max 320 mg/day) | | |
| Oxprenolol + cyclopenthiazide (co-prenozide) | Trasidrex | Tablet | 160 mg + 250 mcg | 1 tablet mane (max 2 tablets mane) | | See also cyclopenthiazide |
| Pindolol | Visken | Tablet | 5, 15 mg | 5 mg 2–3 times/day increasing to 15–30 mg/day (max 45 mg/day) | Contraindicated in asthma, chronic obstructive pulmonary disease, heart block; accumulates in renal impairment (reduce dose); caution in hepatic impairment, pregnancy and breast feeding | Bradycardia, heart failure, conduction disorders, bronchospasm, peripheral vasoconstriction, gastrointestinal effects, fatigue, sleep disturbance |
| Pindolol + clopamide | Viskaldix | Tablet | 10 + 5 mg | 1–2 tablets mane (max 3 mane) | | |
| Propranolol | Inderal | Tablet | 10, 40, 80 mg | 80 mg 2 times/day; maintenance 160–320 mg/day | Contraindicated in asthma, chronic obstructive pulmonary disease and heart block; caution in renal and hepatic impairment, pregnancy and breast feeding; M/R formulations should be swallowed whole | Bradycardia, heart failure, conduction disorders, bronchospasm, peripheral vasoconstriction, gastrointestinal effects, fatigue, sleep disturbance |
| | Half-Inderal LA | M/R capsule | 80 mg | 80–160 mg/day | | |
| | Inderal LA | M/R capsule | 160 mg | 160–320 mg/day | | |

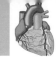

| Drug | Trade name | Preparation | Strength | Doses used in hypertension (adult) | Comments | Side effects |
|---|---|---|---|---|---|---|
| **Beta-adrenoceptor blocking drugs** | | | | | | |
| Propranolol + bendroflu-methiazide | Inderetic | Capsule | 80 + 2.5 mg | 1 capsule 2 times/day | | See also bendroflumethiazide |
| | Inderex | M/R capsule | 160 + 5 mg | 1 capsule/day | | |
| Timolol | Betim | Tablet | 10 mg | 10 mg/day (max 60 mg/day in divided doses if above 20 mg) | Contraindicated in asthma, chronic obstructive pulmonary disease and heart block; caution in renal and hepatic impairment, pregnancy and breast feeding | Bradycardia, heart failure, conduction disorders, bronchospasm, peripheral vasoconstriction, gastrointestinal effects, fatigue, sleep disturbance |
| Timolol + amiloride + hydrochloro-thiazide | Moducren | Tablet | 10 + 2.5 + 25 mg | 1–2 tablets mane | | See also amiloride and hydrochlorothiazide |
| Timolol + bendroflu-methiazide | Prestim | Tablet | 10 + 2.5 mg | 1–2 tablets mane (max 4 tablets mane) | | See also bendroflumethiazide |
| **Vasodilator antihypertensive drugs** | | | | | | |
| Hydralazine | Apresoline | Tablet | 25 mg | 25 mg 2 times/day increasing to 50 mg 2 times/day prn | Contraindicated in idiopathic systemic lupus erythematosus, severe tachycardia, high output heart failure, myocardial insufficiency due to mechanical obstruction, cor pulmonale, dissecting aortic aneurysm, porphyria; caution in hepatic and renal impairment, pregnancy and breast feeding | Tachycardia, palpitations, flushing, fluid retention, gastrointestinal effects |
| Minoxidil | Loniten | Tablet | 2.5, 5, 10 mg | 5 mg/day (2.5 mg/day elderly) (max 50 mg/day) | Contraindicated in phaeochromocytoma; caution in pregnancy | Sodium and water retention, weight gain, peripheral oedema, tachycardia, hypertrichosis |

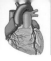

## Centrally acting antihypertensive drugs

| Drug | Trade name | Preparation | Strength | Doses used in hypertension (adult) | Comments | Side effects |
|------|-----------|-------------|----------|-------------------------------------|----------|--------------|
| Clonidine | Catapres | Tablet | 100, 300 mcg | 50–100 mcg 3 times/day (max 1.2 mg/day) | Withdraw gradually to avoid hypertensive crisis | Dry mouth, sedation, depression, fluid retention, bradycardia, occlusive peripheral vascular disease, headache, dizziness, euphoria, rash, nausea, constipation |
| Methyldopa | Aldomet | Tablet | 250, 500 mg | 250 mg 2–3 times/day (125 mg 2 times/day elderly) (max 2 g/day) | Contraindicated in depression, active liver disease, phaeochromocytoma, porphyria; caution in hepatic and renal impairment | Gastrointestinal effects, dry mouth, stomatitis, bradycardia, exacerbation of angina, postural hypotension, oedema, sedation, headache, dizziness, myalgia, arthralgia, nightmares, depression, hepatitis, jaundice, pancreatitis, haemolytic anaemia, bone marrow depression, hypersensitivity reactions, myocarditis, pericarditis, rashes |
| Moxonidine | Physiotens | Tablet | 200, 300, 400 mcg | 200 mcg mane increasing to 400 mcg (max 600 mcg in 2 divided doses) | Contraindicated in conduction disorders, history of angio-oedema, bradycardia, severe heart failure, severe coronary artery disease, unstable angina, pregnancy and breast feeding; caution in severe hepatic or renal impairment | Dry mouth, headache, fatigue, dizziness, nausea, sleep disturbance, asthenia, vasodilatation |

## Alpha-adrenoceptor blocking drugs

| Drug | Trade name | Preparation | Strength | Doses used in hypertension (adult) | Comments | Side effects |
|------|-----------|-------------|----------|-------------------------------------|----------|--------------|
| Doxazosin | Cardura | Tablet | 1, 2 mg | 1 mg/day initially, increasing to 2 mg and 4 mg/day prn (max 16 mg/day) | Contraindicated in urinary incontinence; caution in hepatic impairment | Postural hypotension, dizziness, vertigo, headache, fatigue, asthenia, oedema, somnolence, nausea, rhinitis |
| | Cardura XL | M/R tablet | 4, 8 mg | 4mg/day, increasing to 8mg/day prn (max 8mg/day) | | |

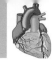

## Alpha-adrenoceptor blocking drugs

| Drug | Trade name | Preparation | Strength | Doses used in hypertension (adult) | Comments | Side effects |
|------|-----------|-------------|----------|-----------------------------------|----------|--------------|
| Indoramin | Baratol | Tablet | 25 mg | 25 mg 2 times/day initially (max 200 mg in 2–3 divided doses) | Contraindicated in urinary incontinence and established heart failure; caution in hepatic and renal impairment | Sedation, dizziness, depression, failure of ejaculation, dry mouth, nasal congestion, extrapyramidal effects, weight gain |
| Prazosin | Hypovase | Tablet | 0.5, 1, 2 mg | 1 mg 2–3 times/day (max 20 mg/day) | Contraindicated in urinary incontinence and congested heart failure; reduce dose in hepatic and renal impairment; caution in pregnancy and breast feeding | Postural hypotension, drowsiness, weakness, dizziness, headache, lack of energy, nausea, palpitations, urinary frequency, incontinence, priapism |
| Terazosin | Hytrin | Tablet | 1, 2, 5, 10 mg | 1 mg nocte increasing to 2–10 mg/day (max 20 mg) | Contraindicated in urinary incontinence | Postural hypotension, dizziness, lack of energy, peripheral oedema, urinary frequency, priapism |

## Angiotensin-converting enzyme inhibitors

| Drug | Trade name | Preparation | Strength | Doses used in hypertension (adult) | Comments | Side effects |
|------|-----------|-------------|----------|-----------------------------------|----------|--------------|
| Captopril | Capoten | Tablet | 12.5, 25, 50 mg | 12.5 mg 2 times daily (6.25 mg 2 times daily with diuretic, elderly) increasing to 25 mg 2 times daily (max 150 mg) | Contraindicated in renovascular disease, aortic stenosis, outflow tract obstruction, porphyria and pregnancy; caution in renal impairment | Renal impairment, persistent dry cough, angio-oedema, rash, pancreatitis, upper respiratory tract effects, gastrointestinal effects, liver function abnormalities, headache, dizziness, fatigue, malaise, taste disturbance, myalgia, arthralgia, tachycardia, serum sickness, weight loss, stomatitis, photosensitivity, flushing |
| Captopril + hydrochloro-thiazide (co-zidocapt) | Capozide LS | Tablet | 25 + 12.5 mg | 1 tablet/day | For mild/moderate hypertension in patients controlled by the individual components in the same proportions | See also hydrochlorothiazide |
| | Capozide | Tablet | 50 + 25 mg | 1 tablet/day | | |

## Angiotensin-converting enzyme inhibitors

| Drug | Trade name | Preparation | Strength | Doses used in hypertension (adult) | Comments | Side effects |
|------|-----------|-------------|----------|-----------------------------------|----------|--------------|
| Cilazapril | Vascace | Tablet | 500 mcg, 1, 2.5, 5 mg | 1 mg/day (500 mcg/day with diuretic, renal impairment, elderly), maintenance 2.5–5 mg/day (max 5 mg/day) | Contraindicated in renovascular disease, aortic stenosis, outflow tract obstruction, severe hepatic impairment and pregnancy; caution in renal impairment | Renal impairment, persistent dry cough, angio-oedema, rash, pancreatitis, upper respiratory tract effects, gastrointestinal effects, liver function abnormalities, headache, dizziness, fatigue, malaise, taste disturbance, myalgia, arthralgia, dyspnoea, bronchitis |
| Enalapril | Innovace | Tablet | 2.5, 5, 10, 20 mg | 5 mg/day (2.5 mg/day with diuretic, renal impairment, elderly), maintenance 10–20 mg/day (max 40 mg/day) | Contraindicated in renovascular disease, aortic stenosis, outflow tract obstruction, porphyria and pregnancy; caution in renal and hepatic impairment | Renal impairment, persistent dry cough, angio-oedema, rash, pancreatitis, upper respiratory tract effects, gastrointestinal effects, liver function abnormalities, headache, dizziness, fatigue, malaise, taste disturbance, myalgia, arthralgia, palpitations, arrhythmias, chest pain, syncope, cerebrovascular accident, anorexia, stomatitis, dermatological effects, confusion, depression, nervousness, insomnia, impotence |
| Enalapril + hydrochlorothiazide | Innozide | Tablet | 20 + 12.5 mg | 1 tablet/day | For mild/moderate hypertension in patients controlled by the individual components in the same proportions | See also hydrochlorothiazide |
| Fosinopril | Staril | Tablet | 10, 20 mg | 10 mg/day (less with diuretic), maintenance 10–40 mg/day (max 40 mg/day) | Contraindicated in renovascular disease, aortic stenosis, outflow tract obstruction, severe hepatic impairment, porphyria and pregnancy; caution in renal impairment | Renal impairment, persistent dry cough, angio-oedema, rash, pancreatitis, upper respiratory tract effects, gastrointestinal effects, liver function abnormalities, headache, dizziness, fatigue, malaise, taste disturbance, myalgia, arthralgia, chest pain, musculoskeletal pain |

## Angiotensin-converting enzyme inhibitors

| Drug | Trade name | Preparation | Strength | Doses used in hypertension (adult) | Comments | Side effects |
|---|---|---|---|---|---|---|
| Imidapril | Tanatril | Tablet | 5, 10, 20 mg | 5 mg/day (2.5 mg/day with diuretic, heart failure cerebrovascular disease, angina, renal or hepatic impairment, elderly), maintenance 10 mg/day (max 20 mg/day) | Contraindicated in renovascular disease, aortic stenosis, outflow tract obstruction and pregnancy; caution in renal and hepatic impairment | Renal impairment, persistent dry cough, angio-oedema, rash, pancreatitis, upper respiratory tract effects, gastrointestinal effects, liver function abnormalities, headache, dizziness, fatigue, malaise, taste disturbance, myalgia, arthralgia, dry mouth, glossitis, abdominal pain, bronchitis, sleep disturbances, depression, confusion, blurred vision, tinnitus, impotence |
| Lisinopril | Carace | Tablet | 2.5, 5, 10, 20 mg | 2.5 mg/day (less with diuretic), maintenance 10–20 mg/day (max 40 mg/day) | Contraindicated in renovascular disease, aortic stenosis, outflow tract obstruction and pregnancy; caution in renal impairment | Renal impairment, persistent dry cough, angio-oedema, rash, pancreatitis, upper respiratory tract effects, gastrointestinal effects, liver function abnormalities, headache, dizziness, fatigue, malaise, taste disturbance, myalgia, tachycardia, cerebrovascular accident, myocardial infarction, dry mouth, confusion, mood changes, asthenia, sweating, impotence |
|  | Zestril | Tablet | 2.5, 5, 10, 20 mg |  |  |  |
| Lisinopril + hydrochloro-thiazide | Carace Plus | Tablet | 10 + 12.5 mg, 20 + 12.5 mg | 1 tablet/day | For mild/moderate hypertension in patients controlled by the individual components in the same proportions | See also hydrochlorothiazide |
|  | Zestoretic | Tablet | 10 + 12.5 mg, 20 + 12.5 mg | 1 tablet/day |  |  |

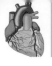

## Angiotensin-converting enzyme inhibitors

| Drug | Trade name | Preparation | Strength | Doses used in hypertension (adult) | Comments | Side effects |
|------|-----------|-------------|----------|-----------------------------------|----------|--------------|
| Moexipril | Perdix | Tablet | 7.5, 15 mg | 7.5 mg/day (3.75 mg/day with diuretic, renal or hepatic impairment, elderly), maintenance 15–30 mg/day (max 30 mg/day) | Contraindicated in renovascular disease, aortic stenosis, outflow tract obstruction and pregnancy; caution in renal and hepatic impairment | Renal impairment, persistent dry cough, angio-oedema, rash, pancreatitis, upper respiratory tract effects, gastrointestinal effects, liver function abnormalities, headache, dizziness, fatigue, malaise, taste disturbance, myalgia, tachycardia, arrhythmias, angina, chest pain, syncope, cerebrovascular accident, myocardial infarction, appetite and weight changes, dry mouth, photosensitivity, flushing, nervousness, mood changes, anxiety, drowsiness, sleep disturbance |
| Perindopril | Coversyl | Tablet | 2, 4, 8 mg | 2 mg/day (less with diuretic), maintenance 4 mg/day (max 8 mg/day) | Contraindicated in renovascular disease, aortic stenosis, outflow tract obstruction and pregnancy; caution in renal and hepatic impairment | Renal impairment, persistent dry cough, angio-oedema, rash, pancreatitis, upper respiratory tract effects, gastrointestinal effects, liver function abnormalities, headache, dizziness, fatigue, malaise, taste disturbance, myalgia, tachycardia, asthenia, flushing, mood and sleep disturbances |
| Perindopril + indapamide | Coversyl Plus | Tablet | 4 + 1.25 mg | 1 tablet/day | | See also indapamide |

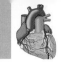

## Angiotensin-converting enzyme inhibitors

| Drug | Trade name | Preparation | Strength | Doses used in hypertension (adult) | Comments | Side effects |
|------|-----------|-------------|----------|-----------------------------------|----------|--------------|
| Quinapril | Accupro | Tablet | 5, 10, 20, 40 mg | 10 mg/day (2.5 mg with diuretic, renal impairment, elderly), maintenance 20–40 mg/day (max 80 mg/day) | Contraindicated in renovascular disease, aortic stenosis, outflow tract obstruction and pregnancy; caution in renal and hepatic impairment | Renal impairment, persistent dry cough, angio-oedema, rash, pancreatitis, upper respiratory tract effects, gastrointestinal effects, liver function abnormalities, headache, dizziness, fatigue, malaise, taste disturbance, myalgia, tachycardia, asthenia, chest pain, oedema, flatulence, nervousness, insomnia, blurred vision, impotence, back pain, myalgia |
| Quinapril + hydrochlorothiazide | Accuretic | Tablet | 10 + 12.5 mg | 1 tablet/day | For mild/moderate hypertension in patients controlled by the individual components in the same proportions | See also hydrochlorothiazide |
| Ramipril | Tritace | Tablet | 1.25, 2.5, 5, 10 mg | 1.25 mg/day (less with diuretic), maintenance 2.5–5 mg/day (max 10 mg/day) | Contraindicated in renovascular disease, aortic stenosis, outflow tract obstruction and pregnancy; caution in renal and hepatic impairment | Renal impairment, persistent dry cough, angio-oedema, rash, pancreatitis, upper respiratory tract effects, gastrointestinal effects, liver function abnormalities, headache, dizziness, fatigue, malaise, taste disturbance, myalgia, tachycardia, arrhythmias, angina, chest pain, myocardial infarction, loss of appetite, dry mouth, dermatological effects, confusion, nervousness, depression, anxiety, impotence, bronchitis, muscle cramps |
| Ramipril + felodipine | Triapin Mite | Tablet | 2.5 + 2.5 mg | 1 tablet/day | For hypertension in patients controlled by the individual components in the same proportions | See also felodipine |
| | Triapin | Tablet | 5 + 5 mg | 1 tablet/day | | |

## Angiotensin-converting enzyme inhibitors

| Drug | Trade name | Preparation | Strength | Doses used in hypertension (adult) | Comments | Side effects |
|------|-----------|-------------|----------|-----------------------------------|----------|--------------|
| Trandolapril | Gopten | Capsule | 500 mcg, 1, 2 mg | 500 mcg/day (less with diuretic), maintenance 1–2 mg/day (max 4 mg/day) | Contraindicated in renovascular disease, aortic stenosis, outflow tract obstruction and pregnancy; caution in renal and hepatic impairment | Renal impairment, persistent dry cough, angio-oedema, rash, pancreatitis, upper respiratory tract effects, gastrointestinal effects, liver function abnormalities, headache, dizziness, fatigue, malaise, taste disturbance, myalgia, tachycardia, arrhythmias, angina, chest pain, cerebral haemorrhage, myocardial infarction, dry mouth, dermatological effects, asthenia, alopecia, dyspnoea, bronchitis |
| | Odrik | Capsule | 500 mcg, 1, 2 mg | | | |
| Trandolapril + verapamil | Tarka | Capsule | 2 + 180 mg | 1 capsule/day | For hypertension in patients controlled by the individual components in the same proportions | See also verapamil |

## Angiotensin II receptor antagonists

| Drug | Trade name | Preparation | Strength | Doses used in hypertension (adult) | Comments | Side effects |
|------|-----------|-------------|----------|-----------------------------------|----------|--------------|
| Candesartan | Amias | Tablet | 2, 4, 8, 16 mg | 4 mg/day (2 mg in hepatic and renal impairment), maintenance 8 mg/day (max 16 mg/day) | Contraindicated in pregnancy and breast feeding; caution in aortic or mitral valve stenosis, obstructive hypertrophic cardiomyopathy, renal and hepatic impairment | Symptomatic hypotension, hyperkalaemia, upper respiratory tract symptoms, abdominal pain, back pain, arthralgia, myalgia, nausea, headache, dizziness, peripheral oedema, rash |
| Eprosartan | Teveten | Tablet | 300, 400, 600 mg | 600 mg/day (300 mg/day >75 years, hepatic and renal impairment), maintenance 800 mg/day | Contraindicated in pregnancy and breast feeding; caution in aortic or mitral valve stenosis, obstructive hypertrophic cardiomyopathy, renal and hepatic impairment | Symptomatic hypotension, hyperkalaemia, flatulence, dizziness, arthralgia, rhinitis, hypertriglyceridaemia |
| Irbesartan | Aprovel | Tablet | 75, 150, 300 mg 150 + 12.5, 300 + 12.5 mg | 150 mg/day (75 mg/day >75 years), maintenance 300 mg/day | Contraindicated in pregnancy and breast feeding; caution in aortic or mitral valve stenosis, obstructive hypertrophic cardiomyopathy, renal and hepatic impairment | Symptomatic hypotension, hyperkalaemia, diarrhoea, dyspepsia, flushing, tachycardia, dizziness, asthenia, myalgia, rash, urticaria |

## Angiotensin II receptor antagonists

| Drug | Trade name | Preparation | Strength | Doses used in hypertension (adult) | Comments | Side effects |
|---|---|---|---|---|---|---|
| Irbesartan + hydrochloro-thiazide | CoAprovel | Tablet | 150 + 12.5, 300 + 12.5 mg | 1 tablet/day | For hypertension in patients controlled by the individual components in the same proportions | See also hydrochlorothiazide |
| Losartan | Cozaar | Tablet | 25, 50, 100 mg | 50 mg/day (25 mg/day >75 years, severe renal impairment) (max 100 mg/day) | Contraindicated in pregnancy and breast feeding; caution in aortic or mitral valve stenosis, obstructive hypertrophic cardiomyopathy, renal and hepatic impairment | Symptomatic hypotension, hyperkalaemia, diarrhoea, dizziness, taste disturbance, cough, myalgia, migraine, urticaria, pruritus, rash |
| Losartan + hydrochloro-thiazide | Cozaar Comp | Tablet | 50 + 12.5 mg | 1 tablet/day | For hypertension in patients controlled by the individual components in the same proportions | See also hydrochlorothiazide |
| Olmesartan | Olmetec | Tablet | 10, 20, 40 mg | 10 mg/day increasing to 20 mg/day prn (max 40 mg/day) | Contraindicated in hepatic impairment, biliary obstruction; pregnancy and breast feeding; caution in aortic or mitral valve stenosis, obstructive hypertrophic cardiomyopathy, renal impairment | Abdominal pain, diarrhoea, dyspepsia, nausea, influenza-like symptoms, cough, pharyngitis, rhinitis, dizziness, haematuria, urinary tract infection, peripheral oedema, arthritis, musculoskeletal pain |
| Telmisartan | Micardis | Tablet | 20, 40, 80 mg | 40 mg/day (max 80 mg/day) | Contraindicated in biliary obstruction, gastric or duodenal ulceration, pregnancy and breast feeding; caution in aortic or mitral valve stenosis, obstructive hypertrophic cardiomyopathy, renal and hepatic impairment | Symptomatic hypotension, hyperkalaemia, gastrointestinal effects, pharyngitis, back pain, myalgia |
| Telmisartan + hydrochlorothiazide | Micardis Plus | Tablet | 40 + 12.5, 80 + 12.5 mg | 1 tablet/day | | See also hydrochlorothiazide |

## Angiotensin II receptor antagonists

| Drug | Trade name | Preparation | Strength | Doses used in hypertension (adult) | Comments | Side effects |
|---|---|---|---|---|---|---|
| Valsartan | Diovan | Capsule | 40, 80, 160 mg | 80 mg/day (40 mg/day >75 years, renal and hepatic impairment) (max 160 mg/day) | Contraindicated in biliary obstruction, cirrhosis, pregnancy and breast feeding; caution in aortic or mitral valve stenosis, obstructive hypertrophic cardiomyopathy, renal and hepatic impairment | Symptomatic hypotension, hyperkalaemia, fatigue |

## Calcium-channel blockers

| Drug | Trade name | Preparation | Strength | Doses used in hypertension (adult) | Comments | Side effects |
|---|---|---|---|---|---|---|
| Amlodipine | Istin | Tablet | 5, 10 mg | 5 mg/day (max 10 mg/day) | Contraindicated in cardiogenic shock, unstable angina, aortic stenosis, pregnancy and breast feeding; caution in renal and hepatic impairment | Headache, oedema, fatigue, nausea, flushing, dizziness, gum hyperplasia, rashes |
| Diltiazem | Adizem-SR | M/R capsule | 90, 120, 180 mg | 120 mg 2 times/day (max 180 mg 2 times/day) | Contraindicated in severe bradycardia, second or third degree atrioventricular block, sick sinus syndrome, pregnancy and breast feeding; reduce dose in hepatic or renal failure or significantly impaired left ventricular function, bradycardia, first degree atrioventricular block or prolonged PR interval; patients should be maintained on the same brand because of variations in clinical effect; all formulations should be swallowed whole; do not use with beta-adrenoceptor blocking drugs | Bradycardia, sino-atrial block, atrioventricular block, palpitations, dizziness, symptomatic hypotension, malaise, asthenia, headache, hot flushes, gastrointestinal effects, constipation, oedema |
| | | M/R tablet | 120 mg | | | |
| | Adizem-XL | M/R capsule | 120, 180, 240, 300 mg | 240 mg/day (120 mg/day elderly, renal and hepatic impairment) (max 300 mg/day) | | |
| | Angitil SR | M/R capsule | 90, 120, 180 mg | 90 mg 2 times/day increasing to 120 mg 2 times/day prn (max 180 mg 2 times/day) | | |
| | Angitil XL | M/R capsule | 240, 300 mg | 240 mg/day (max 300 mg/day) | | |

## Calcium-channel blockers

| Drug | Trade name | Preparation | Strength | Doses used in hypertension (adult) | Comments | Side effects |
|---|---|---|---|---|---|---|
| Diltiazem cont.. | Calcicard CR | M/R tablet | 90, 120 mg | 90–120 mg 2 times/day (120 mg/day elderly, hepatic and renal impairment) (max 360 mg/day) | Contraindicated in severe bradycardia, second or third degree atrioventricular block, sick sinus syndrome, pregnancy and breast feeding; reduce dose in hepatic or renal failure or significantly impaired left ventricular function, bradycardia, first degree atrioventricular block or prolonged PR interval; patients should be maintained on the same brand because of variations in clinical effect; all formulations should be swallowed whole; do not use with beta-adrenoceptor blocking drugs | Bradycardia, sino-atrial block, atrioventricular block, palpitations, dizziness, symptomatic hypotension, malaise, asthenia, headache, hot flushes, gastrointestinal effects, constipation, oedema |
| | Dilcardia SR | M/R capsule | 60, 90, 120 mg | 90 mg 2 times/day (60 mg 2 times/day elderly, hepatic and renal impairment) (max 180 mg 2 times/day) | | |
| | Dilzem SR | M/R capsule | 60, 90, 120 mg | 90 mg 2 times/day (60 mg 2 times/day elderly) (max 180 mg 2 times/day) | | |
| | Dilzem XL | M/R capsule | 120, 180, 240 mg | 180 mg/day (120 mg/day elderly, renal and hepatic impairment) (max 360 mg/day) | | |
| | Slozem | M/R capsule | 120, 180, 240, 300 mg | 240 mg/day (120 mg/day elderly, renal and hepatic impairment) (max 360 mg/day) | | |

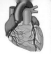

## Calcium-channel blockers

| Drug | Trade name | Preparation | Strength | Doses used in hypertension (adult) | Comments | Side effects |
|---|---|---|---|---|---|---|
| Diltiazem cont.. | Tildiem LA | M/R capsule | 200, 300 mg | 200 mg/day, maintenance 300–400 mg/day (max 500 mg/day, elderly, renal and hepatic impairment 200–300 mg/day) | Contraindicated in severe bradycardia, second or third degree atrioventricular block, sick sinus syndrome, pregnancy and breast feeding; reduce dose in hepatic or renal failure or significantly impaired left ventricular function, bradycardia, first degree atrioventricular block or prolonged PR interval; patients should be maintained on the same brand because of variations in clinical effect; all formulations should be swallowed whole; do not use with beta-adrenoceptor blocking drugs | Bradycardia, sino-atrial block, atrioventricular block, palpitations, dizziness, symptomatic hypotension, malaise, asthenia, headache, hot flushes, gastrointestinal effects, constipation, oedema |
| | Tildiem Retard | M/R tablet | 90, 120 mg | 90–120 mg 2 times/day (120 mg/day elderly, hepatic or renal impairment), (max 360 mg/day in divided doses) | | |
| | Viazem XL | M/R capsule | 120, 180, 240, 300, 360 mg | 180 mg/day (120 mg/day elderly, renal and hepatic impairment) (max 360 mg/day) | | |
| | Zemtard | M/R capsule | 120, 180, 240, 300 mg | 180–300 mg/day (120 mg/day elderly, renal and hepatic impairment) (max 360 mg/day) | | |
| Felodipine | Plendil | M/R tablet | 2.5, 5, 10 mg | 5 mg mane (2.5 mg mane elderly), maintenance 5–10 mg mane (max 20 mg mane) | Contraindicated in unstable angina, uncontrolled heart failure, aortic stenosis, within 1 month of myocardial infarction and pregnancy; caution in renal and hepatic impairment; swallow whole | Flushing, headache, palpitations, dizziness, fatigue, gravitational oedema |

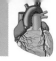

## Calcium-channel blockers

| Drug | Trade name | Preparation | Strength | Doses used in hypertension (adult) | Comments | Side effects |
|---|---|---|---|---|---|---|
| Isradipine | Prescal | Tablet | 2.5 mg | 2.5 mg 2 times/day (1.25 mg 2 times/day elderly, hepatic or renal impairment), maintenance 2.5–10 mg/day (max 10 mg 2 times/day) | Contraindicated in tight aortic stenosis, sick sinus syndrome and pregnancy; caution in renal and hepatic impairment | Headache, flushing, dizziness, tachycardia, palpitations, localized peripheral oedema |
| Lacidipine | Motens | Tablet | 2, 4 mg | 2 mg mane, maintenance 4 mg mane (max 6 mg mane) | Contraindicated in aortic stenosis, within 1 month of myocardial infarction, pregnancy and breast feeding; caution in renal and hepatic impairment | Headache, flushing, oedema, dizziness, palpitations |
| Lercanidipine | Zanidip | Tablet | 10 mg | 10 mg/day (max 20 mg/day; max may be 40 mg in the USA) | Contraindicated in aortic stenosis, unstable angina, uncontrolled heart failure, within 1 month of myocardial infarction and pregnancy; caution in renal and hepatic impairment, left ventricular dysfunction, sick sinus syndrome; take before food | Flushing, peripheral oedema, palpitations, tachycardia, headache, dizziness, asthenia |
| Nicardipine | Cardene | Capsule | 20, 30 mg | 20 mg 3 times/day, maintenance 60–120 mg/day | Contraindicated in cardiogenic shock, aortic stenosis, unstable angina, within 1 month of myocardial infarction, pregnancy and breast feeding; caution in congestive heart failure, impaired left ventricular function, renal and hepatic impairment; M/R formulation should be swallowed whole | Dizziness, headache, peripheral oedema, flushing, palpitations, nausea |
| | Cardene SR | M/R capsule | 30, 45 mg | 30 mg 2 times/day, maintenance 30–60 mg 2 times/day | | |

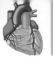 
## Calcium-channel blockers

| Drug | Trade name | Preparation | Strength | Doses used in hypertension (adult) | Comments | Side effects |
|---|---|---|---|---|---|---|
| Nifedipine | Adalat LA | M/R tablet | 20, 30, 60 mg | 20–30 mg/day (max 90 mg/day) | Contraindicated in cardiogenic shock, advanced aortic stenosis, unstable angina, within 1 month of myocardial infarction, porphyria; caution in pregnancy and breast feeding, congestive heart failure, impaired left ventricular function, renal and hepatic impairment; patients should be maintained on the same brand because of variations in clinical effect; all formulations should be swallowed whole | Headache, flushing, dizziness, lethargy, tachycardia, palpitations, gravitational oedema, rash, pruritus, urticaria, nausea, constipation, visual disturbances, gum hyperplasia, paraesthesia, impotence, depression |
| | Adalat Retard | M/R tablet | 10, 20 mg | 10 mg 2 times/day (max 40 mg 2 times/day) | | |
| | Adipine MR | M/R tablet | 10, 20 mg | 10 mg 2 times/day (max 40 mg 2 times/day) | | |
| | Cardilate MR | M/R tablet | 10, 20 mg | 10 mg 2 times/day (max 80 mg/day) | | |
| | Coracten SR | M/R capsule | 10, 20 mg | 20 mg 2 times/day, maintenance 10–40 mg 2 times/day | | |
| | Coracten XL | M/R capsule | 30, 60 mg | 30 mg/day (max 90 mg/day) | | |
| | Coroday MR | M/R tablet | 20 mg | 20 mg 2 times/day (max 40 mg 2 times/day) | | |
| | Fortipine LA 40 | M/R tablet | 40 mg | 40 mg/day (max 80 mg/day) | | |
| | Hyolar Retard 20 | M/R tablet | 20 mg | 20 mg 2 times/day (max 40 mg 2 times/day) | | |
| | Nifedipress MR | M/R tablet | 10 mg | 10 mg 2 times/day (max 40 mg 2 times/day) | | |

## Calcium-channel blockers

| Drug | Trade name | Preparation | Strength | Doses used in hypertension (adult) | Comments | Side effects |
|------|-----------|-------------|----------|-----------------------------------|----------|-------------|
| Nifedipine cont... | Nifopress Retard | M/R tablet | 20 mg | 20 mg 2 times/day (max 40 mg 2 times/day) | Contraindicated in cardiogenic shock, advanced aortic stenosis, unstable angina, within 1 month of myocardial infarction, porphyria; caution in pregnancy and breast feeding, congestive heart failure, impaired left ventricular function, renal and hepatic impairment; patients should be maintained on the same brand because of variations in clinical effect; all formulations should be swallowed whole | Headache, flushing, dizziness, lethargy, tachycardia, palpitations, gravitational oedema, rash, pruritus, urticaria, nausea, constipation, visual disturbances, gum hyperplasia, paraesthesia, impotence, depression |
| | Slofedipine | M/R tablet | 20 mg | 20 mg 2 times/day (max 40 mg 2 times/day) | | |
| | Slofedipine XL | M/R tablet | 30, 60 mg | 30 mg/day (max 90 mg/day) | | |
| | Tersipine MR | M/R tablet | 10, 20 mg | 10 mg 2 times/day (max 40 mg 2 times/day) | | |
| Nisoldipine | Syscor MR | M/R tablet | 10, 20, 30 mg | 10 mg daily (max 40 mg daily) | Contraindicated in cardiogenic shock, aortic stenosis, unstable angina, within 1 month of myocardial infarction, hepatic impairment; pregnancy and breast feeding; caution in renal impairment; swallow whole | Gravitational oedema, headache, flushing, tachycardia, palpitations, dizziness, asthenia, gastrointestinal effects |

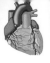

## Calcium-channel blockers

| Drug | Trade name | Preparation | Strength | Doses used in hypertension (adult) | Comments | Side effects |
|---|---|---|---|---|---|---|
| Verapamil | Cordilox | Tablet | 40, 80, 120, 160 mg | 240–480 mg/day in 2–3 divided doses | Contraindicated in bradycardia, second or third degree atrioventricular block, sick sinus syndrome, cardiogenic shock, sino-atrial block, impaired left ventricular function, porphyria; caution in first degree atrioventricular block, acute phase of myocardial infarction, hepatic impairment, pregnancy and breast feeding; do not use with beta-adrenoceptor blocking drugs; M/R formulations should be swallowed whole | Constipation, nausea, vomiting, flushing, headache, dizziness, fatigue, ankle oedema |
| | Securon | Tablet | 40, 120 mg | | | |
| | Half Securon SR | M/R tablet | 120 mg | 120 mg/day, maintenance | | |
| | Securon SR | M/R tablet | 240 mg | 240 mg/day (max 480 mg/day) | | |
| | Univer | M/R capsule | 120, 180, 240 mg | 240 mg/day (max 480 mg/day) | | |
| | Verapress MR | M/R tablet | 240 mg | 1 tablet/day (max 1 tablet 2 times/day) | | |
| | Vertab SR 240 | M/R tablet | 240 mg | 1 tablet/day (max 1 tablet 2 times/day) | | |

# Abbreviations

## Drugs

| | |
|---|---|
| AIIRA | Angiotensin II receptor antagonist |
| COC | Combined oral contraceptive |
| HRT | Hormone replacement therapy |
| NSAID | Non-steroidal anti-inflammatory drug |

## Examinations and procedures

| | |
|---|---|
| ABPM | Ambulatory blood pressure monitoring |
| BMI | Body mass index |
| CPAP | Continuous positive airways pressure |
| CT | Computed tomography |
| ECG | Electrocardiogram |
| ESR | Erythrocyte sedimentation rate |
| MRI | Magnetic resonance imaging |

## Molecules

| | |
|---|---|
| ACE | Angiotensin-converting enzyme |
| ACTH | Adrenocorticotropin hormone |
| COX-1 | Cyclo-oxygenase type 1 |
| COX-2 | Cyclo-oxygenase type 2 |
| $HbA_{1c}$ | Glycosylated haemoglobin |
| HDL | High-density lipoprotein |
| LDL | Low-density lipoprotein |
| MIBG | Metaiodobenzylguanidine |
| VMA | Vanillyl mandelic acid |

## Organizations

| | |
|---|---|
| BHS | British Hypertension Society |
| ESC | European Society of Cardiology |
| ESH | European Society of Hypertension |
| JNC7 | The Seventh Report of the Joint National Committee on prevention, detection, evaluation, and treatment of high blood pressure |
| MRC | Medical Research Council |

## Other

| | |
|---|---|
| CHD | Coronary heart disease |
| ISA | Intrinsic sympathomimetic activity |
| ISH | Isolated systolic hypertension |
| LVH | Left ventricular hypertrophy |
| MI | Myocardial infarction |

117

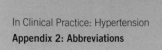
## Trials

| | |
|---|---|
| ALLHAT | Antihypertensive and Lipid-Lowering treatment to prevent Heart Attack Trial |
| ANBP2 | Second Australian National Blood Pressure study |
| ASCOT | Anglo-Scandinavian Cardiovascular Outcomes Trial |
| BPLTTC | Blood Pressure Lowering Treatment Trialists Collaboration |
| HOT | Hypertension Optimal Treatment |
| HYVET | Hypertension in the Very Elderly Trial |
| LIFE | Losartan Intervention For Endpoint reduction in hypertension |
| PROGRESS | Perindopril Protection Against Recurrent Stroke Study |
| SHEP | Systolic Hypertension in the Elderly Program |
| Syst-Eur | Systolic Hypertension in Europe |
| TOMHS | Treatment of Mild Hypertension Study |
| UKPDS | United Kingdom Prospective Diabetes Study |

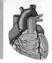

# Contact information for useful organizations

## For the health professional

### American College of Cardiology
Heart House, 9111 Old Georgetown Road, Bethesda, MD 20814-1699, USA
Tel: 800 253 4636, ext. 694
Fax: 301 897 9745
Website: http://www.acc.org

### American Diabetes Association
(Attn: National Call Center), 1701 North Beauregard Street,
Alexandria, VA 22311, USA
Tel: 800 342 2383
Website http://www.diabetes.org

### American Heart Association
One North Franklin, Chicago, IL 60606-3412, USA
Tel: 312 422 3000
Website: http://www.aha.org

### American Society of Hypertension
148 Madison Avenue, New York, NY 10016, USA
Tel: 212 696 9099
Fax: 212 696 0711
E-mail: ash@ash-us.org

### American Stroke Association
National Center, 7272 Greenville Avenue, Dallas, TX 75231, USA
Tel: 800 242 8721
Website: http://www.strokeasscociation.org

### Blood Pressure Association
60 Cranmer Terrace, London SW17 0QS, UK
Tel: 020 8772 4994
Fax: 020 8772 4999
Website: http://www.bpassoc.org.uk

### British Cardiac Society
9 Fitzroy Square, London W1T 5HW, UK
Tel: 020 7383 3887
Fax: 020 7388 0903

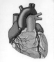

Website: http://www.bcs.com

### British Hypertension Society
Blood Pressure Unit, Department of Physiological Medicine, St George's Hospital Medical School, Cranmer Terrace, London SW17 0RE, UK
Tel: 020 8725 3412
Fax: 020 8725 2959
E-mail: bhsis@sghms.ac.uk
Website: http://www.hyp.ac.uk/bhs

### Consensus Action on Salt and Health (CASH)
Blood Pressure Unit, Department of Medicine, St George's Hospital Medical School, London SW17 0RE, UK
Tel: 020 8725 2409
E-mail: cash@sghms.ac.uk
Website: http://www.hyp.ac.uk/cash/

### Diabetes UK
10 Parkway, London NW1 7AA, UK
Tel: 020 7424 1000
Fax: 020 7424 1001
E-mail: info@diabetes.org.uk
Website: http://www.diabetes.org.uk

### European Atherosclerosis Society
Secretary, Dr Sebastiano Calandra, Sezione di Patologia Generale, Dipartimento di Scienze Biomediche, Universita di Modena e Reggio Emilia, Via Campi 287, I-41100 Modena, Italy
Tel: (+39) 059 2055 423
Fax: (+39) 059 2055 426
Website: http://www.elsevier.com/inca

### European Society of Cardiology
The European Heart House, 2035 Route des Colles B.P. 179 – Les Templiers, FR-06903 Sophia Antipolis, France
Tel: (+33) 4 92 94 76 00
Fax: (+33) 4 92 94 76 01
E-mail: webmaster@escardio.org
Website: http://www.escardio.org

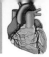

### European Society of Hypertension

Institute of Clinical Experimental Medicine, Dept of Preventive
Cardiology, Videnska 1958/9. 140 21 Prague 4. Czech Republic
Tel: (+420) 2 617 11 399
Fax: (+420) 2 617 10 666
E-mail: info@eshonline.org
Website: http://www.eshonline.org

### International Society of Hypertension in Blacks

2045 Manchester Street, NE Atlanta, Georgia 30324, USA
Tel: 404 875 6263
Website: http://www.ishib.org/

### World Hypertension League

Website: http://www.mco.edu/org/whl/

## For the patient

### American Diabetes Association

(see above)

### British Heart Foundation

14 Fitzhardinge Street, London W1H 6DH, UK
Tel: 020 7935 0185
Fax: 020 7486 5820
E-mail: internet@bhf.org.uk
Website: http://www.bhf.org.uk

### Diabetes UK

(see above)

### Heart UK

7 North Road, Maidenhead, Berkshire SL6 1PE, UK
Tel: 01628 628 638
Fax: 01628 628 698
E-mail: ask@heartuk.org.uk
Website: http://www.heartuk.org.uk

### Life Clinic

Website: http://www.lifeclinic.com/focus/blood/default.asp

# References

1. Collins R, MacMahon S. Blood pressure, antihypertensive drug treatment and risk of stroke and coronary heart disease. Br Med Bull 1994;50:272–98.
2. Prospective Studies Collaboration. Age-specific relevance of usual blood pressure to vascular mortality: a meta-analysis of individual data one million adults in 61 studies. Lancet 2002;360:1903–13.
3. Kearney PM, Whelton M, Reynolds K et al. Worldwide prevalence of hypertension: a systematic review. J Hypertens 2004;22:11–19.
4. Andersson OK, Almgren T, Persson B et al. Survival in treated hypertension: follow up study after two decades. BMJ 1998;317:167–71.
5. Guidelines Committee. 2003 European Society of Hypertension – European Society of Cardiology guidelines for the management of arterial hypertension. J Hypertens 2003;21;1011–53. (http://www.eshonline.org/documents/2003_guidelines.pdf)
6. Chobanian AV, Bakris GL, Black HR et al. The Seventh Report of the Joint National Committee on prevention, detection, evaluation, and treatment of high blood pressure. The JNC 7 report. JAMA 2003;289:2560–72; revised fuller version, Hypertension 2003;42:1206.
7. Nawrot T, Den Hond E, Thijs L et al. Isolated systolic hypertension and the risk of vascular disease. Curr Hypertens Rep 2003;5:372–9.
8. British Hypertension Society website: http://www.hyp.ac.uk/bhs/home.htm
9. Bulpitt CJ, Fletcher AE, Amery A et al. Hypertension in the Very Elderly Trial: protocol for the main trial. Drugs Aging 2001;18:151–64.
10. Lever AF, Lyall F, Morton JJ et al. Angiotensin II, vascular structure and blood pressure. Kidney Int 1992;37(Suppl):S51–5.
11. Mulvany MJ. Small artery remodeling and significance in the development of hypertension. News Physiol Sci 2002;17:105–9.
12. Staessen JA, Wang J, Bianchi G et al. Essential hypertension. Lancet 2003;361:1629–41.
13. De Wardener HE, MacGregor GA. Sodium and blood pressure. Curr Opin Cardiol 2002;17:360–7.
14. Mackenzie IS, Brown MJ. Genetic profiling versus drug rotation in the optimisation of antihypertensive treatment. Clin Med 2002;2:465–73.
15. Barker DJ. Fetal programming of coronary heart disease. Trends Endocrinol Metab 2002;13:264–8.
16. Sowers JR. Obesity as a cardiovascular risk factor. Am J Med 2003;115(8A):37S–41S.
17. Isomaa B. A major health hazard: the metabolic syndrome. Life Sci 2003;73:2395–411.
18. Bloomgarden ZT. Obesity, hypertension, and insulin resistance. Diabetes Care 2002;25:2088–97.
19. Pickering T. Cardiovascular pathways: socioeconomic status and stress effects on hypertension and cardiovascular function. Ann NY Acad Sci 1999;896:262–77.
20. Steptoe A, Feldman PJ, Kunz S et al. Stress responsivity and socioeconomic status: a mechanism for increased cardiovascular risk? Eur Heart J 2002;23:1757–63.
21. Poulter NR, Khaw KT, Hopwood BE et al. The Kenyan Luo migration study: observations on the initiation of a rise in blood pressure. BMJ 1990;300:967–72.
22. Safian RD, Textor SC. Renal-artery stenosis. N Engl J Med 2001;344:431–42.
23. Bloch MJ, Basile J. The diagnosis and management of renovascular disease: a primary care perspective. Part II. Issues in management. J Clin Hypertens 2003;5:261–8.
24. Young WF. Minireview: primary aldosteronism-changing concepts in diagnosis and treatment. Endocrinology 2003;144:2208–13.
25. Bravo EL, Tagle R. Pheochromocytoma: state-of-the-art and future prospects. Endocrine Revs 2003;24:539–663.
26. Shamsuzzaman ASM, Gersh BJ, Somers VK. Obstructive sleep apnea. Implications for cardiac and vascular disease. JAMA 2003;290:1906–14.
27. Chaturvedi N. Ethnic differences in cardiovascular disease. Heart 2003;89:681–6.
28. Morley Kotchen J, Kotchen TA. Impact of female hormones on blood pressure: review of potential mechanisms and clinical studies. Curr Hypertens Rep 2003;5:505–12.
29. Meune C, Mourad JJ, Bergmann JF et al. Interaction between cyclooxygenase and the renin-angiotensin-aldosterone system: rationale and clinical relevance. J Renin Angiotensin Aldosterone Syst 2003;4:149–54.
30. Fowles RE. Potential cardiovascular effects of COX-2 selective nonsteroidal antiinflammatory drugs. J Pain Palliat Care Pharmacother 2003;17:27–50.
31. Curtis JJ. Hypertensinogenic mechanisms of the calcineurin inhibitors. Curr Hypertens Rep 2002;4:377–80.
32. Smith KJ, Bleyer AJ, Little WC et al. The cardiovascular effects of erythropoietin. Cardiovasc Res 2003;59:538–48.
33. Brennelsen R, Fisch HU, Koelbing U et al. Amphetamine-like effects in humans of the khat alkaloid cathinone. Br J Clin Pharmacol 1990;30:825–8.
34. Klingbeil AU, Schneider M, Martus P et al. A meta-analysis of the effects of treatment on left ventricular mass in essential hypertension. Am J Med 2003;115:41–6.
35. Liebson PR. Left ventricular hypertrophy in hypertension. 2. Results of clinical trials of regression. Heart Drug 2002;2:251–65.
36. Vakili BA, Okin PM, Devereux RB. Prognostic implications of left ventricular hypertrophy. Am Heart J 2001;141:334–41.
37. Lip GY. Hypertension and the prothrombotic state. J Hum Hypertens 2000;14:687–90.

38. Manolio TA, Olson J, Longstreth WT. Hypertension and cognitive function: pathophysiological effects of hypertension on the brain. Curr Hypertens Reps 2003;5:255–61.

39. Leys D. Neurological protection provided by candesartan: reviewing the latest study results. Curr Med Res Opin 2003;19:445–8.

40. Mogensen CE. Microalbuminuria and hypertension with focus on type 1 and 2 diabetes. J Intern Med 2003;254:45–66.

41. Verdecchia P, Angeli F, Gattobigio R. Clinical usefulness of ambulatory blood pressure monitoring. J Am Soc Nephrol 2004;15(Suppl 1):S30–3.

42. Padwal R, Li SK, Lau DC. Long-term pharmacotherapy for overweight and obesity: systematic review and meta-analysis of randomized controlled trials. Int J Obes Relat Metab Disord 2003;27:1437–46.

43. Williams B, Poulter NR, Brown MJ et al. British Hypertension Society guidelines for hypertension management 2004 (BHS-IV): summary. BMJ 2004;328:634–40. (for full version: J Hum Hypertens 2004;18:139–85.)

44. Berlowitz DR, Ash AS, Hickey EC et al. Inadequate management of blood pressure in a hypertensive population. N Engl J Med 1998;339:1957–63.

45. Wolf-Maier K, Cooper RS, Kjramer H et al. Hypertension treatment and control in five European countries, Canada, and the United States. Hypertension 2004;43:10–7.

46. Hosie J, Wiklund I. Managing hypertension in general practice: can we do better? J Hum Hypertens 1995;9(Suppl 2):S15–8.

47. Jones JK, Gorkin L, Lian JF et al. Discontinuation of and changes in treatment after start of new courses of antihypertensive drugs: a study of a United Kingdom population. BMJ 1995;311:293–5.

48. Bloom BS. Continuation of initial antihypertensive medication after 1 year of therapy. Clin Ther 1998;20:671–81.

49. Neaton DJ, Grimm RH, Prineas RJ et al. Treatment of Mild Hypertension Study (TOMHS): final results. JAMA 1993;270:713–24.

50. Materson BJ, Reda DJ, Cushman WC et al. Single-drug therapy for hypertension in men. A comparison of six antihypertensive agents with placebo. The Department of Veterans Affairs Cooperative Study Group on Antihypertensive Agents. N Engl J Med 1993;328:914–21.

51. Gibbs CR, Beevers DG, Lip GY. The management of hypertensive disease in black patients. QJM 1999;92:187–92.

52. Psaty BM, Lumley T, Furberg CD et al. Health outcomes associated with various antihypertensive therapies used as first-line agents. A network meta-analysis. JAMA 2003;289:2534–44.

53. ALLHAT Officers and Coordinators for the ALLHAT Collaborative Research Group. Major outcomes in high-risk hypertensive patients randomized to angiotensin-converting enzyme inhibitor or calcium channel blocker vs diuretic: The Antihypertensive and Lipid-Lowering Treatment to Prevent Heart Attack Trial (ALLHAT). JAMA 2002;288:2981–97. See also Medscape website for continuing debate: http://www.medscape.com/pages/editorial/resourcecenters/public/allhat/rc-allhat.ov

54. Wing LM, Reid CM, Ryan P et al. A comparison of outcomes with angiotensin-converting-enzyme inhibitors and diuretics for hypertension in the elderly. N Engl J Med 2003;348:583–92.

55. Stewart JR, Yeun JY. Initial therapy for uncomplicated hypertension: insights from the alphabetic maze of recent studies. Minerva Med 2003;94:2315–27.

56. Chalmers JP, Arnolda LF. Lowering blood pressure in 2003. MJA 2003;179:306–12.

57. Brown MJ, Cruickshank JK, Dominiczak AF et al. Better blood pressure control: how to combine drugs. J Human Hypertens 2003;17:81–6.

58. Hansson L, Zanchetti A, Carruthers SG et al. Effects of intensive blood pressure lowering and low dose aspirin in patients with hypertension: principal results of the Hypertension Optimised Therapy (HOT) randomised trial. Lancet 1998;351:1755–62.

59. United Kingdom Prospective Diabetes Study group. Tight blood pressure control and risk of microvascular and macrovascular complications in type 2 diabetes. UKPDS 38. BMJ 1998;317:703–17.

60. Schachter M. New approaches in the treatment of hypertension. In: Kaplan NM, Schachter M, editors. New Frontiers in Hypertension. London: Lippincot Williams and Wilkins, 2002;pp.101–13.

61. PROGRESS Collaborative Group. Randomised trial of a perindopril-based blood-pressure-lowering regimen among 6105 individuals with previous stroke or transient ischaemic attack. Lancet 2001;358:1033–41.

62. Law MR, Wald NJ, Morris JK et al. Value of low dose combination treatment with blood pressure lowering drugs: analysis of 354 randomised trials. BMJ 2003;326:1427–34.

63. Neutel JM, Smith DH. The circadian pattern of blood pressure: cardiovascular risks and therapeutic opportunities. Curr Opin Nephrol Hypertens 1997;6:250–6.

64. Mancia G, Parati G. Importance of smooth and sustained blood pressure control in preventing cardiovascular morbidity and mortality. Blood Press 2001;3(Suppl):26–32.

65 White WB. Cardiovascular risk and therapeutic intervention for the early morning surge in blood pressure and heart rate. Blood Press Monit 2001;6:63–72.

66. Sica DA, White W. Chronotherapeutics and its role in the treatment of hypertension and cardiovascular disease. J Clin Hypertens 2000;2:279–86.

67. Tsai P-S. White coat hypertension: understanding the concept and examining the significance. J Clin Nurs 2002;11:715–22.

68. Wing LM, Brown MA, Beilin LJ et al. "Reverse white coat hypertension" in older hypertensives. J Hypertens 2002;20:639–44.

69. SHEP Cooperative Research Group. Prevention of stroke by antihypertensive drug treatment in older persons with isolated systolic hypertension. Final results of the Systolic Hypertension in the Elderly Program (SHEP). JAMA 1991;265:3255–64.

70. Staessens JA, Fargard R, Thijs L et al. Randomised double-blind comparison of placebo and active treatment for older patients with isolated systolic hypertension, The Systolic Hypertension in Europe (Syst-Eur) Investigators. Lancet 1997;350:757–64.

71. Dahlöf B, Devereux RB, Kjeldsen SE et al. Cardiovascular morbidity and mortality in the Losartan Intervention For Endpoint reduction in hypertension study: a randomised trial against atenolol. Lancet 2002;359:995–1003.

72. Moser M. Treatment of hypertension in the very elderly: a clinician's point of view. J Clin Hypertens 2003;5:310–2.

73. Frohlich ED, Sowers JR. Management of diabetic and hypertensive cardiovascular disease. Curr Hypertens Rep 2003;5:309–15.

74. Abrahamson MJ. Clinical use of thiazolidinediones: recommendations. Am J Med 2003;115(Suppl 8A):116S–20S.

75. Hollenberg NK. Considerations for management of fluid dynamics issues associated with thiazolidinediones. Am J Med 2003;115(Suppl 8A):111S–5S.

76. Grossman E, Messerli FH. Are calcium antagonists beneficial in diabetic patients with hypertension? Am J Med 2004;116:44–9.

77. Borghi C, Esposti DD, Cassani A et al. The treatment of hypertension in pregnancy. J Hypertens 2002;20(Suppl 2):S52–6.

78. Vidt DG. Pathogenesis and treatment of resistant hypertension. Minerva Med 2003;94:201–14.

79. Nishizaka MK, Zaman MA, Calhoun DA. Efficacy of low-dose spironolactone in subjects with resistant hypertension. Am J Hypertens 2003;15:925–30.

80. Phillips RA, Greenblatt J, Krakoff LR. Hypertensive emergencies: diagnosis and treatment. Progr Cardiovasc Dis 2002;45:33–48.

81. Shayne PH, Pitts SR. Severely increased blood pressure in the emergency department. Ann Emerg Med 2003;41:513–29.

82. Wald NJ, Law MR. A strategy to reduce cardiovascular disease by more than 80%. BMJ 2003;325:1419.

83. Sever PS, Dahlof B, Poulter NR et al. Anglo-Scandinavian Cardiac Outcomes Trial: a brief history, rationale and outline protocol. J Hum Hypertens 2001;15(Suppl 1):S11–2.

84. Blood Pressure Lowering Treatment Trialists' Collaboration. Effects of ACE inhibitors, calcium antagonists, and other blood-pressure-lowering drugs: results of prospectively designed overviews of randomised trials. Lancet 2002;355:1955–64.

85. The Blood Pressure Lowering Treatment Trialists' Collaboration – second cycle of analyses. Online: http://www.medscape.com/viewarticle/457831

86. McInnes GT. The differences between ACE inhibitor-treated and calcium channel blocker-treated hypertensive patients. J Clin Hypertens 2003;5:337–44.

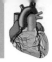

# Index

**Notes:** Abbreviations used in this index are the same as those listed on pages 117-118. As the subject of this book is hypertension, all entries refer to this unless otherwise indicated. Page numbers in *italics* refer to figures or tables.

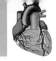

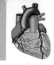

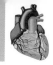

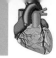

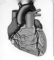